W9-DEE-637

BREAST DISEASE

DIAGNOSIS AND TREATMENT

From the Annual Meeting of
The Society for the Study of Breast Disease
Philadelphia, Pa.
1980

BREAST
DISEASE
DIAGNOSIS AND TREATMENT

EDITORS

GORDON F. SCHWARTZ, M.D.

Professor of Surgery, Jefferson Medical College;
Director of Clinical Services, Breast Diagnostic Center,
Thomas Jefferson University Hospital, Philadelphia, Pa.

DOUGLAS MARCHANT, M.D.

Professor of Obstetrics and Gynecology,
Tufts University School of Medicine;
Director, The Cancer Center,
Tufts-New England Medical Center,
Boston, Mass.

Published by

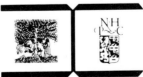

Symposia Specialists Inc.

MEDICAL BOOKS

Distributed by

ELSEVIER/NORTH-HOLLAND
NEW YORK • AMSTERDAM • OXFORD

VANDERBILT UNIVERSITY
MEDICAL CENTER LIBRARY

MAY 21 1982

NASHVILLE, TENNESSEE
37232

Published by:

Symposia Specialists, Inc.
1470 N.E. 129th Street, Miami, Florida 33161

Distributed by:

Elsevier North Holland, Inc.
52 Vanderbilt Avenue, New York, New York 10017

Sole distributors outside U.S.A. and Canada

Elsevier Science Publishers B.V.
P.O. Box 211
1000 AE Amsterdam
The Netherlands

©1981 by Symposia Specialists, Inc.

Library of Congress Catalog Card Number 81-51628
International Standard Book Number 0-444-0593-5

Manufactured in the United States of America

Contents

PHYSIOLOGY AND PATHOLOGY OF BREAST DISEASE

Arthur S. Patchefsky, M.D.
Department of Pathology
Jefferson Medical College
Thomas Jefferson University
Philadelphia, Pa.

John P. Minton, M.D., Ph.D.
Department of Surgery
Ohio State University College of Medicine
Columbus

BREAST CANCER – TREATMENT AND PRETREATMENT CONSIDERATIONS

Gary S. Shaber, M.D.
Department of Radiology
Breast Diagnostic Center
Thomas Jefferson University Hospital
Philadelphia, Pa.

Barbara S. Hulka, M.D., M.P.H.
Department of Epidemiology
University of North Carolina
Chapel Hill

Henry Patrick Leis, Jr., M.D.
Department of Surgery
New York Medical College
Valhalla

Sven J. Kister, M.D.
Department of Surgery
College of Physicians and Surgeons
Columbia University
New York, N.Y.

BREAST CANCER – POSTTREATMENT CONSIDERATIONS

Introduction

Although carcinoma of the breast is the most common cause of cancer death in women and accounts for 28% of all malignancies, the majority of lesions are benign. Pain, nipple discharge and fibrocystic changes continue to account for more than 70% of the problems requiring diagnosis and treatment.

The obstetrician/gynecologist, often the primary physician for women, is frequently consulted for the diagnosis and treatment of benign conditions. Family physicians are concerned with the identification of high-risk patients. Surgeons, aware of newer concepts in the biology of breast cancer, more readily accept alternatives in treatment, including modified radical mastectomy and primary radiotherapy.

This volume represents discussions from the Fourth Annual Meeting of The Society for the Study of Breast Disease, Philadelphia, April 18-20, 1980. They provide an overview of the physiology, detection, diagnosis and treatment of a variety of breast diseases. Many of the papers represent original contributions. Some are controversial. All are written by experts in their fields. Each of the articles presents the objectives of the author and each is accompanied by a self-assessment quiz.

I am particularly grateful to Rose Kushner, Executive Director of the Women's Breast Cancer Advisory Center and member of the National Cancer Advisory Board, who with the help of transparencies provided by Vincent DeVita and Marc Lippman of the National Cancer Institute, presented an excellent overview of "the state of the art for the 80's." Her final message places the problem in perspective: "Women still hope that a cure for breast cancer will be found. We will settle for a way to prevent it: a vaccine, a special diet or whatever. For now we are reconciled to hoping for control. If we can be kept free of symptoms by a few pills a day with little or no side effects, we will wait for the rest."

Founded as the Gynecologic Society for the Study of Breast Disease in 1976, the Society is a multidisciplinary organization representing physicians, medical scientists and nurses. The Society participated in the Fifth Congress of the International Society of Senology, Hamburg, Germany. It was active in the planning of the Sixth Congress held in Barcelona, Spain,May 25-29, 1981; and was co-sponsor of the Nineteenth National Conference on Breast Cancer in San Diego, March 9-13, 1981.

The editors are grateful to the contributors for their prompt response in reviewing the manuscripts prepared from the recorded material presented at the Conference.

Douglas J. Marchant, M.D.
President, The Society for the Study of Breast Disease

Diagnosis of Breast Disease — Benign and Malignant

Low-Dose Mammography: Estimation of the Hypothetical Risk

Stephen A. Feig, M.D.

Objectives

The purpose of this paper is to discuss our present knowledge of mammographic risk and benefit. Hopefully, it will dispel some misconceptions regarding mammography and encourage further appropriate use of this procedure. Tissue dosage from current mammographic technique is below one rad and no excess breast cancer has been observed in this low-dose range. If there is a risk at these levels, it is extremely small and the upper limits of its numerical value can be estimated from high-dose effects such as those seen in atomic bomb survivors. This hypothetical risk is practically negligible when compared to the substantial number of breast cancers detected by mammography at an early, curable stage.

Historically speaking, the great advances in medicine have been those which altered the occurrence or outcome of a major disease. In this context, mammography may be among them. Certainly, its ability to detect carcinoma at a relatively early, preclinical stage, prior to lymph node metastases, would suggest that its widespread use could substantially reduce breast cancer mortality.

Some examples of carcinoma detected on mammography which could not be palpated on physical examination are shown in Figures 1 and 2. Overall, among self-selected women screened

Stephen A. Feig, M.D., Professor of Radiology, Jefferson Medical College; Chief, Section of Mammography, Department of Radiology, Thomas Jefferson University Hospital, Philadelphia, Pa.

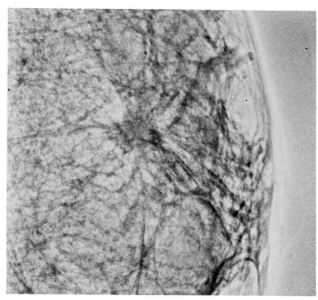

FIG. 1. Invasive ductal carcinoma seen as a 1.0-cm stellate mass on xeromammography. Physical examination was negative. Patient had no symptoms or signs of breast cancer. Axillary nodes showed no evidence of metastatic disease on pathological examination. (Reprinted from Feig [1], ©1979, American Medical Association.)

at the 27 NCI-ACS-supported Breast Cancer Detection Demonstration Projects, where physical examination and mammography were each interpreted with no knowledge of findings from the other modality, only 56% (330/593) of cancers were found by physical examination on initial screening (Fig. 3). Among 460 cancers associated with negative lymph nodes, only 50% (230/460) were detected on physical examination, whereas 93% (428/460) were detected on mammography [1].

Although mammography is frequently employed in clinical practice, the fact that it has not come into even wider use is mainly due to an unnecessary fear concerning the extremely small hypothetical risk which may be associated with low doses of radiation. Though the exposure dose from mammography has been reduced 8- to 20-fold over the past several years [2], many women and their physicians are still gripped by a common ailment known as mammography phobia. The causes

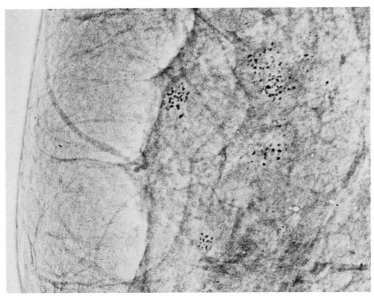

FIG. 2. Nonpalpable clusters of microcalcifications observed on xeromammography were shown to be multiple foci of minimally invasive ductal carcinoma on pathological examination. Axillary nodes were normal. (Reprinted from Feig [1], ©1979, American Medical Association.)

of this malady are ignorance and irrationality. The end results are the unnecessary deaths of women whose cancers are detected too late for curative therapy.

Excess Risk Found in Female Study Populations Exposed to High Doses of Radiation

The breast cancer risk from very low doses of radiation, such as those used in current mammographic techniques, if in fact it does exist, is so extremely small that it has never been directly measured in human populations exposed to low doses of gamma radiation. Its possible existence has only been inferred from the excess cancer incidence observed in groups of women exposed to high doses when they were compared to comparable groups of nonexposed women. These were:

1. Japanese survivors of the atomic bombings at Hiroshima and Nagasaki [3].

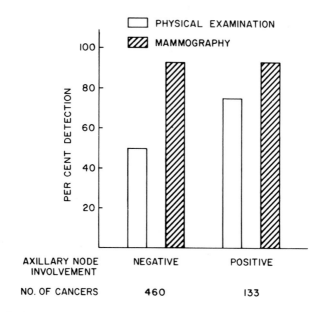

FIG. 3. Detection of 593 cancers on initial screening at the BCDDP by mammography and physical examination according to lymph node status. (Reprinted from Feig [1], © 1979, American Medical Association.)

2. Women from Rochester, New York, treated with radiotherapy for postpartum mastitis [4].
3. Swedish women who received radiation therapy for a variety of benign breast conditions, such as fibroadenomas and mastitis [5].
4. Nova Scota sanitoria patients [6-8].
5. Massachusetts sanitoria patients [9].

The last two groups were monitored by multiple fluoroscopic examinations of the chest during treatment for pulmonary tuberculosis.

Is There Risk at Low Doses?

Because the doses received were relatively high (Rochester, Sweden, Nova Scotia) or an insufficient number of women were exposed to low doses (Japan, Massachusetts), these studies provide little or no useful information regarding the possible effect of low doses of x-rays on the breast. (X-rays are gamma radiation produced by an x-ray machine. Otherwise, the terms may be used synonymously.)

For example, the lowest average dose to both breasts in the Rochester radiotherapy series was 112 rads (Fig. 4). (Actually, since only one third of the women received treatment to both breasts, the lowest mean dose per breast was even higher at 150 rads.) In the Nova Scotia fluoroscopy series, the lowest mean estimated dose was 261 rads (Fig. 5). These breast tissue doses were several hundredfold greater than those obtained from current low-dose mammographic techniques, which range from 0.1 to 0.8 rad [2].

Although these human studies provide few significant data on the low-dose region (below 25 rads), some useful information can be obtained from animal experiments [10]. These

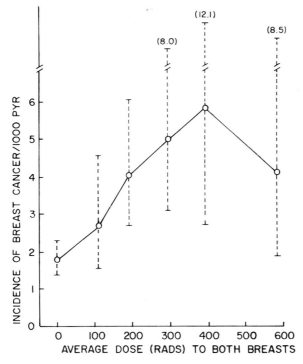

FIG. 4. Relationship of breast cancer incidence to breast tissue dose in Rochester, N.Y., women treated by radiotherapy for postpartum mastitis. (Reprinted from Feig [17], ©1979, Masson Publishing USA, Inc., New York.)

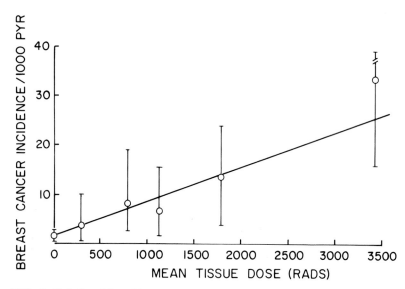

FIG. 5. Relationship of breast cancer incidence to estimated breast tissue
dose from fluoroscopy of Nova Scotia sanitoria patients. (Reprinted from
Feig [17], ©1979, Masson Publishing USA, Inc., New York.)

involve a variety of tumors induced by gamma radiation in
various organs. These experiments usually produce dose-
response curves consisting of three distinct components (Fig. 6).
The mid portion of the curve is a rising straight line. It is linear.
Here, incidence is directly proportional to the first power of
dose; over this part of the curve, effect per rad remains
constant. At high doses, corresponding to the upper portion of
the curve, the slope decreases. Here, effect per rad is less than at
low or medium doses due to cell killing and sterilization.

In nearly all animal models, the lowest portion of the curve
(below 50 or 25 rads) is concave upward. Here, incidence varies
as an exponential function of dose so that effect per rad is less
than expected from downward extrapolation from the higher
dose portion of the curve. In a minority of of animal systems,
the curve continues downward to the origin as a straight line.
One such case might be radiation-induced mammary carcinoma
in the rat (Fig. 7) [11]. On the other hand, if the results are
tabulated in terms of mammary tumors per animal, rather than
the percentage of animals with tumors, a clearly curvilinear
dose-response relationship is seen at low doses (Fig. 8) [12].

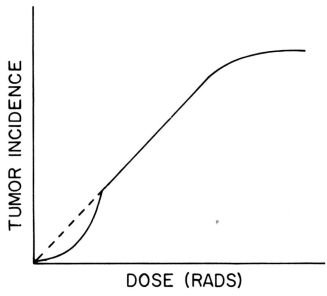

FIG. 6. Dose-response curve for radiation carcinogenesis in animals. (Reprinted from Feig [17], ©1979, Masson Publishing USA, Inc., New York.)

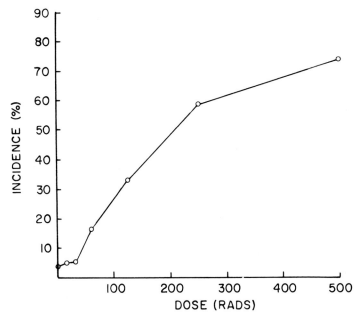

FIG. 7. Percentage of rats with mammary tumors vs. gamma ray dose. (Modified from U.N. Scientific Committee [10].)

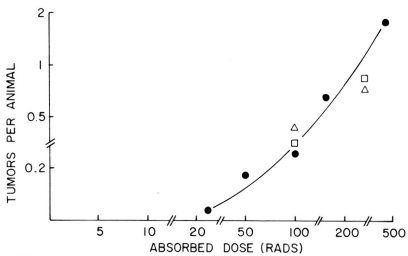

FIG. 8. Breast tumors per rat vs. x-ray dose. (Reprinted from Rossi and Kellerer [12], ©1972, American Association for the Advancement of Science.)

Animal experiments do provide useful qualitiative information which can, by inference, fill the gap in our knowledge that results from lack of human data for the low-dose region. Specifically, one could argue that if low doses of radiation do cause breast cancer, the most likely dose-response-curve shape in that region is curvilinear. In that case, extrapolation downward from the known portion of the human curve would result in an overstatement of risk. On the other hand, one could assume the more conservative linear hypothesis: risk per rad remains constant down at low doses. This latter assumption most probably represents the upper limits of risk. For that reason, it has been used in most risk estimates for human breast cancer.

Assessment of Possible Low-Dose Risk From Female Study Populations

Even assuming the linear hypothesis, the hypothetical risk from low doses is exceedingly small. For women of all ages irradiated in the Western populations (Nova Scotia, Massachusetts, Rochester), it is 7.5 cancers per million women per rad per year [13].

In the Massachusetts fluoroscopy study, no excess cancers were recorded among 395 women in the group with the lowest mean dose of 35 rads (Fig. 9). However, because the estimation of risk is so small, the number of women in this group is not sufficient to exclude the same risk per rad as exists at higher doses. The same is true for a study involving Toronto sanatoria patients where no excess cancers were found among 269 women receiving a mean dose of 17 rads [14].

The Japanese women comprise a larger group, many of whom did receive doses below 100 rads. Analysis of these data is complicated by the fact that Hiroshima women received both gamma and neutron radiation, while the smaller group of Nagasaki survivors received a nearly total gamma dose. For most biological effects in both animals and humans, low doses of neutron radiation have a greater effect per rad than do identical doses of gamma radiation. This effect occurs principally below 50 rads and can be appreciated from Figure 10. Below these doses, the dose-effect curve for gamma radiation becomes

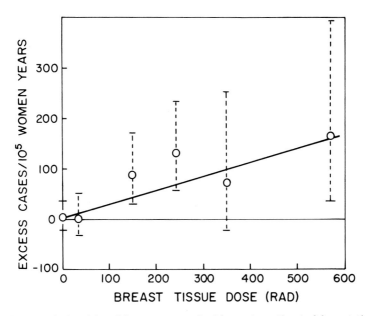

FIG. 9. Relationship of breast cancer incidence to estimated breast tissue dose from fluoroscopy of Massachusetts sanitoria patients. (Reprinted from Feig [18], ©1978, The Chemical Rubber Co., CRC Press, Inc.)

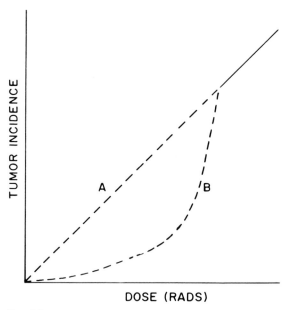

FIG. 10. Possible carcinogenesis at relatively low levels of radiation. Known linear dose-response relationship (solid line) terminates at 25 to 50 rads. Curve A would be expected if the linear hypothesis were valid at low doses. Curve B, which represents a lower risk estimate at low doses, is concave upward with no threshold.

curvilinear (B) while that for neutron radiation remains linear (A). This higher relative biological effect (RBE) is due to the fact that soft tissue ionization from neutrons occurs in a more concentrated manner.

It is not certain if neutrons are more effective than gamma radiation for breast cancer induction in women, but it should be noted that the Hiroshima curve is almost consistently higher than that of Nagasaki (Fig. 11). The difference between the two cities is most marked between 50 and 99 rads. Between 10 and 49 rads the curves appear to approach each other, as do the curves in Figure 10. At the latter doses, curve shape depends on what one accepts as a baseline incidence for naturally occurring breast cancer. There are three possible baselines for each city. These are women exposed at 1 to 9 rads, residents in the city at the time of bombing but unexposed, and residents out of the city at the time of bombing. The number of excess cancers (if

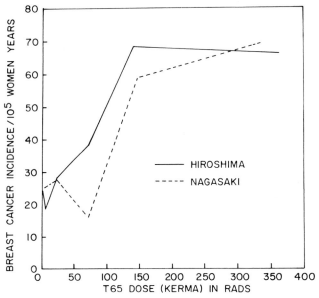

FIG. 11. Relationship of breast cancer incidence to estimated dose in atomic bomb survivors. (Repinted from Feig [17], ©1979, Masson Publishing USA, Inc., New York.)

any) observed will also depend on one's choice of baseline. But in no case, even if all data from both cities including both gamma and neutron radiation are combined, has a statistically significant excess (0.05 level) been shown for doses below 100 rads.

Reduced Risk Estimates for Women
Over 30 Years of Age

There is now abundant evidence that the estimate for the upper limit of possible risk (linear hypothesis) from low doses of radiation is even lower among women over 30 years of age at time of exposure than among younger women. Therefore, it has been possible to lower this risk estimate to a value more appropriate to the older women, on whom mammography might be performed.

Among Japanese women, the risk for those over 35 years of age at time of exposure was less than half that seen in younger women. Dependence of radiation sensitivity on age at time of exposure was also evident among the study populations of Nova Scotia, Sweden and Massachusetts. But since the Japanese population was larger and contained a wider age range than did the others, the National Cancer Institute has used it to obtain a risk adjustment factor of 0.45. When this factor is multiplied by the absolute risk estimate of 7.5 excess cancers per million women per rad per year seen in Western populations, a lowered risk estimate of 3.5 cancers per million women per rad per year is obtained for Western women over 30 years old at time of exposure [13].

The observation that breast sensitivity to radiation declines with patient age represents an epidemiologic finding of major significance since, as can be seen from Figure 13, the incidence of naturally occurring breast cancer increases with patient age. In fact, 97% of naturally occurring breast cancers are found in women over 35 years of age. Therefore, these women would derive the greatest benefit and incur the least risk from mammographic examination.

Latent and Duration Effect

The minimal latent period refers to the time between exposure and appearance of an excess of observed cancers in the irradiated group, compared to those expected from the control group. Figure 12 illustrates determination of the latent period for the Rochester women. For them, as well as for those from Nova Scotia and Massachusetts, the excess did not occur until 15 to 20 years postexposure. The duration of carcinogenic effect is unknown, but all studies indicate that it persists for at least another 15 years. Further follow-up will be necessary to determine its actual length.

Low-Dose Risk Estimate: Comparison with the Natural Breast Cancer Incidence

The extremely small magnitude of possible risk for low-dose mammography can best be appreciated by comparison with the much larger incidence of naturally occurring breast cancer. If one assumes an absolute risk of 3.5 excess cancers per million women per rad per year for those exposed at age 30 or above, then a single mammographic examination with a mean breast

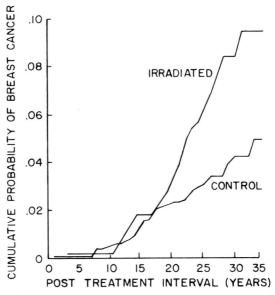

FIG. 12. Determination of latent period for excess breast cancer incidence in Rochester, N.Y., women treated by radiotherapy for postpartum mastitis. (Reprinted from Feig [18], ©1978, The Chemical Rubber Co., CRC Press, Inc.)

dose of 0.3 rad might result in one excess breast cancer per year per million women examined after a latent period of 15 years. This figure can be compared to the much larger natural breast cancer incidence which rises from 1000 cases per million women per year at age 40 to 2000 cases per million women per year at age 70 [15] (Fig. 13). Considering that a substantial portion of these cancers could be detected by mammography at an early, curable stage, the theoretical risk for mammography appears quite negligible.

Verification of Low-Dose Risk Estimate

Can a low-dose risk estimate of 3.5 excess cancers per million women per rad per year be proven or disproven by careful follow-up of women who have received low doses of radiation from mammography? An analogy might be drawn to a situation in which one is trying to hear radio music of gradually diminishing volume in a room with a constant loud background

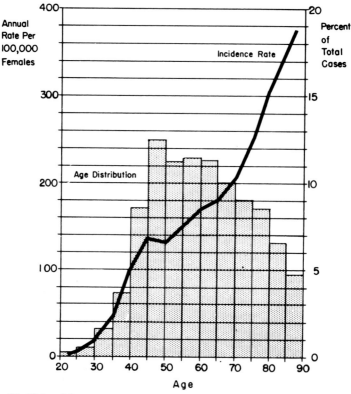

FIG. 13. Natural breast cancer incidence rates and distribution of cases by age. (Reprinted from Seidman [15], ©1972, American Cancer Society.)

noise from a vacuum cleaner or dishwasher. Because the possible low-dose radiation effect is several hundred to thousands of times less than the natural breast cancer incidence, an extremely large population of women would be needed to confirm or deny its existence. Statistical confirmation of a risk of 3.5 cancers per million women per rad per year from an absorbed dose of 1 rad would require 20-year follow-up of 100 million women so exposed, as well as a similar size population of nonexposed women [16].

Further Reduction in Risk Estimates

For two separate reasons, the figure of 3.5 excess cancers per million women per rad per year for women exposed after 30 years of age probably represents an overestimate of risk. First, it is based on the assumption that risk per rad is the same at both high and low doses. Most animal experiments indicate considerably diminished risk per rad at low doses [10].

Second, further analysis of the Nova Scotia, Massachusetts and Swedish studies suggests that radiation risk to women over 30 years of age at time of exposure may be even less than indicated from the Japanese data. Among Massachusetts sanitoria patients 30 years of age or older at time of exposure, no excess breast cancers were demonstrated [9]. Among Nova Scotia patients receiving multiple fluoroscopies and Swedish women treated by radiotherapy for benign breast disease, cancer induction in women over 30 years of age was only 20% of that seen in younger women [5, 8].

Summary

The maximum risk from a single low-dose mammographic exmination with a mean tissue dose of 0.3 rad to women 35 years or older at time of exposure would be one excess cancer per year after a latent period of 15 years. It is likely that the actual risk would be significantly smaller than this figure indicates. Thus, the risk from low-dose mammography is hypothetical and practically negligible, while the benefit is substantial and well documented.

References

1. Feig, S.A.: Low dose mammography. Application to medical practice. JAMA 242:2107-2109, 1979.
2. Muntz, E.P., Wilkinson, E. and George, F.W.: Mammography at reduced doses: Present performance and future possibilities. Am. J. Roentgenol. 134:741-748, 1980.
3. McGregor, D.H., Land, C.E., Choi, K. et al: Breast cancer incidence among atomic bomb survivors, Hiroshima and Nagasaki, 1950-1969. JNCI 59:799-811, 1977.
4. Shore, R.E., Hempelmann, L.H., Kowaluk, E. et al: Breast neoplasms in women treated with x-rays for acute postpartum mastitis. JNCI 59:813-822, 1977.
5. Baral, E., Larsson, L-E. and Mattson, B.: Breast cancer following irradiation of the breast. Cancer 40:2905-2910, 1977.
6. MacKenzie, I.: Breast cancer following multiple fluoroscopies. Br. J. Cancer 19:1-8, 1965.

7. Myrden, J.A. and Hiltz, J.E.: Breast cancer following multiple fluoroscopies during artificial pneuomothorax treatment of pulmonary tuberculosis. Can. Med. Assoc. J. 100:1032-1034, 1969.

8. Myrden, J.A. and Quinlan, J.J.: Breast carcinoma following multiple fluoroscopies with pneumothorax treatment of pulmonary tuberculosis. Ann. R. Coll. Physicians Can. 7:45, 1974.

9. Boice, J.D. and Monson, R.B.: Breast cancer following repeated fluoroscopic examinations of the breast. JNCI 59:823-832, 1977.

10. United Nations Scientific Committee on the Effects of Atomic Radiation: Sources and Effects of Atomic Radiation, 1977 Report to the General Assembly, with annexes. New York:United Nations, 1977.

11. Shellabarger, C.J., Bond, V.P., Cronkite, E.P. et al: Relationship of dose of total body ^{60}Co radiation to incidence of mammary neoplasia in female rats. In Radiation-Induced Cancer, IAEA-SM-118/9. Vienna: International Atomic Energy Agency, 1969, pp. 161-172.

12. Rossi, H. and Kellerer, A.: Radiation carcinogenesis at low doses. Science 175:200-202, 1972.

13. Upton, A.C., Beebe, G.W., Brown, J.M. et al: Report of the NCI Ad Hoc Working Group on the Risks Associated with Mammography in Mass Screening for the Detection of Breast Cancer. JNCI 59:481-493, 1977.

14. Delarue, N.C., Gale, G. and Ronald, A.: Multiple fluoroscopy of the chest: Carcinogenicity for the female breast and implications for breast cancer screening programs. Can. Med. Assoc. J. 112:1405-1411, 1975.

15. Seidman, H.: Cancer of the Breast, Statistical and Epidemiological Data. New York:American Cancer Society, 1972, p. 28.

16. Mammography. Washington:National Council on Radiation Protection and Measurements, 1980. (In press.)

17. Feig, S.A.: Epidemiology of radiation-related breast cancer. In Logan, W.W. and Muntz, E.P. (eds.): Reduced Dose Mammography. New York:Masson Publishing U.S.A., Inc., 1979.

18. Feig, S.A.: Ionizing radiation and human breast cancer, CRC Crit. Rev. Diagn. Imaging 11(2):155, 160, 1978.

Self-Evaluation Quiz

1. At the Breast Cancer Detection Demonstration Projects (BCDDP) the percentage of cancers with negative findings on physical examination was:

    a) 10%

    b) 22%

    c) 38%

    d) 44%

    e) 76%

2. Which of the following were true of the BCDDP results:
   a) 93% of cancers with negative nodes were found on mammography
   b) 50% of cancers with negative nodes were found on physical examination
   c) 95% of cancers with positive nodes were found on mammography
   d) 75% of cancers with positive nodes were found on physical examination
   e) All of the above
3. Evidence that high doses of radiation cause breast cancer has been found in all of the following groups except:
   a) Tuberculosis sanitoria patients
   b) Atomic bomb survivors
   c) Women treated by radiotherapy for mastitis
   d) Women exposed to multiple mammographic examinations
   e) Animal experiments
4. Evidence that doses below 1 rad may cause breast cancer has been:
   a) Directly observed in Japanese A-bomb survivors
   b) Directly observed in sanitoria patients
   c) Directly observed in women exposed to multiple mammographic examinations
   d) Postulated from excess breast cancers seen in women exposed to doses above 100 rads
   e) All of the above
5. Most animal experiments indicate that the effectiveness per rad of low doses of gamma radiation is _____ the effectivenesss per rad of higher doses.
   a) Greater than
   b) Less than
   c) Equal to
6. Which of the following statements are true?
   a) A statistically significant breast cancer increase was not seen in Japanese women receiving less than 100 rads of gamma radiation
   b) Breast tissue doses from current mammographic equipment are generally 0.1 to 0.8 rad
   c) No excess breast cancers were found among Massachusetts sanitoria patients receiving doses of 35 rads

d) No excess breast cancers were found among Toronto sanitoria patients receiving doses of 17 rads

e) All of the above

7. All of the following concerning decreased radiation risk estimates in older women are true *except:*

a) Risk may be half that seen in younger women

b) "Older women" refers to only those above 50 years of age

c) Decreased risk for older women was seen in Nova Scotia, Swedish, Massachusetts and Japanese studies

d) Decreased risk with age is an important observation since older women benefit most from mammographic screening

8. With respect to analysis of possible low-dose effect in Japanese A-bomb survivors, all of the following represent actual shortcomings of the data *except:*

a) No women were exposed to low doses

b) An insufficient number of women were exposed to low doses of gamma radiation

c) Most were exposed to both neutron and gamma radiation

d) Retrospective dosage estimates may not be accurate

e) Choice of a baseline incidence of naturally occurring breast cancers may alter the shape of the dose-response curve

9. At low doses, the graph of breast tumors per rat vs. absorbed dose:

a) Is a straight line

b) Is concave upward

c) Is concave downward

d) Shows a threshold level

10. Concerning radiation carcinogenesis, animal experiments demonstrate all of the following *except:*

a) Neutron radiation is more effective per rad than gamma radiation

b) Dose-response relationship at low doses is exponential

c) An exact quantitative estimate of low-dose risk to humans

d) Cell killing and sterilization at very high doses

11. Following radiation exposure to the breast, the risk of carcinogenic effect shows:
   a) Latent period of 1 year and lifetime duration
   b) Latent period of 1 year and 5-year duration
   c) Latent period of 5 years and 10-year duration
   d) Latent period of 15 years and duration of at least 15 years
   e) Latent period of 25 years and lifetime duration
12. If one million women each received a mean breast tissue dose of 0.3 rad, the number of excess cancers per year after the latent period has been estimated to be:
   a) 1
   b) 5
   c) 20
   d) 50
   e) 1000
13. The number of naturally occurring (nonradiogenic) breast cancers in one million women aged 40 during a period of one year is:
   a) 20
   b) 50
   c) 100
   d) 500
   e) 1000
14. Which of the following are true?
   a) Excess breast cancers were found in Nova Scotia sanitoria patients receiving a mean tissue dose of 100 rads
   b) Excess breast cancers were found among Rochester radiotherapy patients receiving a mean dose per breast of 50 rads
   c) Linear extrapolation of risk from high doses represents the upper limits of risk at low doses
   d) All of the above
   e) None of the above
15. Statistical confirmation of the low-dose risk estimate for humans:
   a) Would require 15-year follow-up of 10,000 women exposed to 1 rad each
   b) Could be obtained from animal experiments

c) Is practically impossible because the risk is extremely small in relation to the natural breast cancer incidence
d) Could be obtained from tissue culture experiments
e) Has been obtained from Japanese A-bomb survivors

Answers on page 335.

Low-Dose Mammography: Assessment of Benefit vs. Risk

Stephen A. Feig, M.D.

Objectives

This paper will review:
1. The proof that decreased breast cancer mortality has resulted from mammographic screening of asymptomatic women above 50 years of age.
2. The evidence that this benefit can be increased and extended to women between 35 and 50 years of age by means of current mammographic techniques.
3. The guidelines for mammographic examination of symptomatic and asymptomatic women provided by the American College of Radiology.

Quantitative assessment of benefit vs. risk is not usually a factor when the clinical physician considers the use of mammography for a woman of any age with symptoms or signs of possible breast cancer. In these instances, he is trying to answer an immediate clinical question, such as whether a breast "lump" appears benign or malignant, or whether biopsy is indicated. Mammography may confirm or refute his initial clinical impression of benign or malignant disease. A negative mammogram may provide reassurance to a concerned patient. In these situations, not all the benefits of mammography can be given numerical value. These types of clinical problems do not lend themselves to a quantitative comparison of benefit vs. risk.

However, benefit/risk ratios can be calculated for mammographic screening of asymptomatic women. Since the hypo-

Stephen A. Feig, M.D., Professor of Radiology, Jefferson Medical College; Chief, Section of Mammography, Department of Radiology, Thomas Jefferson University Hospital, Philadelphia, Pa.

thetical risk from low-dose mammography is of practically negligible magnitude and the ability of mammography to detect breast cancer at an early, nonpalpable stage has been repeatedly demonstrated, it would seem that no one could possibly question the efficacy of mammographic screening for all women in the breast cancer age group (ages 35 to 40 and older).

Although everyone has supported mammographic screening of asymptomatic women above 50 years of age, some have questioned screening asymptomatic women below age 50 [1]. This viewpoint reflects their unwillingness to acknowledge any benefit in screening this younger age group. To them, risk, no matter how infinitesimal, will always exceed benefit if the latter value is equal to zero.

The roots of this attitude may be found in the results of a breast cancer screening program conducted by the Health Insurance Plan of Greater New York between 1963 and 1967 [2]. Sixty-two thousand female volunteers between 40 and 64 years of age were allocated to study and control groups of 31,000 women each. The study group only was offered four annual clinical and mammographic examinations. When breast cancer mortality rates in these two groups were compared, a one-third reduction in breast cancer mortality was found in the study group, compared to the control group (Fig. 1) [3]. However, the entire benefit was confined to women over 50 years of age at the time of detection. Decreased mortality was not shown for younger women. Actually, if only women over 50 years of age at time of detection are considered, decreased mortality in this group would be over 40%. This reduction still persists on the most recent follow-up of nine years (1975).

Although Shapiro, the project statistician, has stated that "a 20-30% reduction in mortality in women below 50 could be missed in a study of this size," one must search for other explanations. One possibility is that the clinical course of breast cancer is different in women above and below age 50. According to this hypothesis, early detection would improve prognosis only in the older age group. This is a poor theory for two reasons. First, review of the medical literature indicates no difference in breast cancer mortality rates according to patient age when similar-stage lesions are compared [4]. Second, for women below 50 years of age, the HIP Project Study Group did

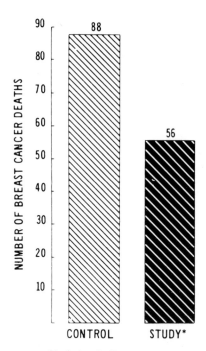

*Includes deaths among women screened and
those who refused screening.

FIG. 1. Thirty-six percent decreased breast cancer mortality among
screened (study) vs. nonscreened (control) women above 50 years of age
was proven in the HIP study. Current data from BCDDP projects suggests
that this gain can be increased in magnitude and extended to women
below 50 years of age. (Reprinted from Venet et al [3], ©1975, John
Wiley & Sons, Inc.)

not contain a significantly greater proportion of cancers with
negative nodes than did the control group [5].

The most plausible reason for the HIP Study's inability to
demonstrate decreased mortality in women below 50 was that
mammographic detection of early cancers was less effective in
that age group. Since the time of that project (1963 to 1967),
there has been a marked improvement in mammographic
equipment and imaging systems as well as diagnostic expertise.
Analysis of more current data from the 27 NCI-ACS-sponsored
Breast Cancer Detection Demonstration Projects [6] suggests
that decreased mortality in women under 50 years of age could

now be demonstrated. These projects were begun in 1973 for five annual clinical and mammographic screenings of 270,000 women between 35 and 74 years of age. Comparison of data from the HIP and BCDDP projects yields several major observations:

1. From the time of HIP to the BCDDP studies, there has been an enormous improvement in the ability of mammography to detect early cancers (defined here as minimal cancers: all infiltrative cancers less than 1 cm and all in situ cancers) in women of all age groups (Table 1). Considering that detection rates on first screening for all cancers at the BCDDP are twice those at the HIP study (5.54 per 1000 vs. 2.73 per 1000), there have been approximately seven times as many minimal cancers detected per 1000 patients screened at the BCDDP as at the HIP study.

2. In the earlier HIP study, mammographic detection was less effective in women below 50 years of age than in older women. In the current BCDDP study, it is equally effective in both age groups (Fig. 2).

3. The HIP study proved that cancers detected by mammography alone have exceptionally low case fatality rates (Table 2). Among women below 50 years of age, there were few such cases in the HIP study (20%) but relatively more (45%) in the BCDDP study (Fig. 2).

4. Among patients with negative axillary lymph nodes in the BCDDP project, 95% were detected by mammography but only 50% by physical examination (see Fig. 3 of previous paper).

Table 1. Detection of Minimal Breast Cancers
for BCDDP (First Two Screenings) and HIP Studies

	HIP	BCCDP
Minimal cancers/total cancers	8% (5/61)	28% (374/1336)
Percent Detection by Modality		
M+,C−	40% (2/5)	65% (244/374)
M+,C+	0% (0/5)	30% (110/374)
M−,C+	60% (3/5)	3% (12/374)
Total M+	40% (2/5)	95% (354/374)

Source: References 5 and 6.

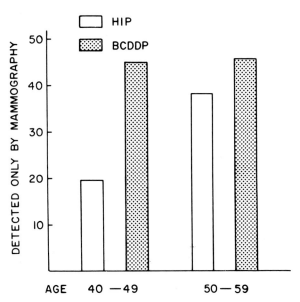

FIG. 2. Percentage of breast cancers detected only by mammography among women ages 40 to 49 and 50 to 59 years. Comparison of results from the HIP study (1963-1967) and the BCDDP projects (1973-1976). (Reprinted from Feig [16], ©1979, American Medical Association.)

The foregoing analysis indicates that mammography had a significant role in effecting the 40% decrease in breast cancer mortality found among women over 50 years of age at time of detection in the HIP study. It strongly suggests that a substantially greater decrease in breast cancer mortality in that age group could result from current mammographic techniques, such as those employed at the BCDDP, and that the decrease in mortality would be extended to those between 35 and 50 years of age at time of detection.

Unlike the HIP project, the BCDDP projects were not conducted in the form of a randomized clinical trial where

Table 2. Breast Cancer Mortality Rates in HIP Study

M+, C+	41%
M−, C+	32%
M+, C−	14%

Source: Shapiro [2].

breast cancer mortality was simultaneously measured in control and study populations. The BCDDP data do indicate that substantially decreased breast cancer mortality through screening with current techniques is a reasonable expectation in women between 35 and 50 years of age, but it does not provide the same degree of proof as would be obtained from a randomized clinical trial [7].

Such proof should be forthcoming from randomized clinical trials now under way in Sweden [8] and Canada [9], but results from these are at least ten years away. In the meantime, the best estimates of benefit from mammographic screening can be found in several rigorous mathematical analyses based on current data from the BCDDP projects. Two of these evaluations yield benefit/risk ratios of approximately 100:1, based on a single initial screening of women between 35 and 50 years of age [10, 11]. Calculations based on five annual screenings produce lower ratios because of lower detection rates, but all strongly support the validity of screening these younger women with low-dose techniques [12-14].

These studies support the American College of Radiology Policy Statement on Mammography [15], which lists the following indications for mammography:

  1. All women with signs or symptoms of possible breast cancer.
  2. Screening of asymptomatic women.
    A. Annual physical examination and periodic breast self-examination.
    B. Baseline mammogram between age 35 and 40.
    C. Subsequent mammography at 1- to 3-year intervals, based on risk factors (more frequent if medically warranted).
    D. After age 50, annual or other regular-interval mammography.

References

1. Bailar, J.C.: Mammography, a contrary view. Ann. Intern. Med. 84:77-84, 1976.
2. Shapiro, S.: Evidence on screening for breast cancer from a randomized trial. Cancer 39:2772-2782, 1977.
3. Venet, L., Shapiro, S., Strax, P. et al: Effect of screening on survival. *In* Gallager, H.S. (ed.): Early Breast Cancer, Detection, and Treatment. New York:John Wiley & Sons, 1975, pp. 97-103.

4. Stoll, B.A.: Effect of age on growth pattern. *In* Stoll, B.A. (ed.): Risk Factors in Breast Cancer. Chicago:Year Book Medical Publishers, 1976.

5. Report of the NCI Ad Hoc Pathology Working Group to Review the Gross and Microscopic Findings of Breast Cancer Cases in the HIP Study (Health Insurance Plan of Greater New York). JNCI 59:497-541, 1977.

6. Beahrs, O.H., Shapiro, S. and Smart, C.: Report of the working group to review the National Cancer Institute-American Cancer Society Breast Cancer Detection Demonstration Projects. JNCI 62:640-709, 1979.

7. Feig, S.A.: Effect of early breast cancer detection, theory and experience. *In* Logan, W.W. and Muntz, E.P. (eds.): Reduced Dose Mammography. New York:Masson Publishing USA, Inc., 1979, pp. 77-95.

8. Tabar, L., Gad, A., Akerlund, B. et al: Screening for breast cancer in Sweden. A randomized clinical trial. *In* Logan, W.W. and Muntz, E.P. (eds.): Reduced Dose Mammography. New York:Masson Publishing USA, Inc., 1979, pp. 407-415.

9. National breast cancer screening study gets under way. Can. Med. Assoc. J. 122:243-244, 1980.

10. Gregg, E.C.: Radiation risk with diagnostic x-rays. Radiology 123:447-452, 1977.

11. Moskowitz, M., Keriakes, J., Saenger, E.L. et al: Breast cancer screening. Benefit and risk for the first annual screening. Radiology 120:431-432, 1976.

12. Chiacchierini, R.P. and Lundin, F.E.: Risk-benefit analysis for reduced dose mammography. *In* Logan, W.W. and Muntz, E.P. (eds.): Reduced Dose Mammography. New York:Masson Publishing USA, Inc., 1979, pp. 61-72.

13. Fox, S.S., Moskowitz, M., Saenger, E.L. et al: Benefit/risk analysis of aggressive mammographic screening. Radiology 128:359-365, 1978.

14. Seidman, H.: Screening for beast cancer in younger women. Life expectancy gains and losses. An analysis according to risk indicator groups. CA 27:66-87, 1977.

15. Board approves mammography policy, summary of current opinion, American College of Radiology. Bull. Am. Coll. Radiol. 32:1, 1976.

16. Feig, S.A.: Low dose mammography. Application to medical practice. JAMA 242:2107-2109, 1979.

Self-Evaluation Quiz

1. Support for screening women below 50 years of age has come from:
   a) HIP study
   b) BCDDP study
   c) Randomized clinical trials in Canada

    d) Randomized clinical trials in Sweden
    e) None of the above
2. Concerning breast cancer detection among women less than 50 years of age in the HIP study:
    a) A 20% to 30% decrease in breast cancer mortality could have been missed due to the limited number of women examined
    b) It proved that early detection does not affect prognosis in younger women
    c) Results are unclear because breast cancer prognosis is normally worse in younger women
    d) All of the above
    e) None of the above
3. Concering the HIP study group:
    a) Decreased mortality was not shown for women below 50 years of age at time of detection
    b) A 40% decreased mortality was shown for women above 50 years of age at time of detection
    c) Cancers detected by mammography alone had exceptionally low case fatality rates
    d) Among women over 50 years of age at time of detection, nearly 40% of cancers were detected by mamography alone; among women below 50 years of age, 20% of cancers were detected by mammography alone
    e) All of the above
4. All of the following BCDDP data support mammographic screening of women below age 50 *except*:
    a) Among cancers with negative axillary nodes, 95% were detected by mammography, 50% by physical examination
    b) Mammographic detection was equally effective among women above and below age 50
    c) In women either below or above age 50, 45% of breast cancers were detected by mammography and not by physical examination
    d) The BCDDP has been conducted as a randomized clinical trial
    e) None of the above
5. A randomized clinical trial:

    a) Compares breast cancer survival rates in study and control populations

    b) Compares breast cancer mortality rates in study and control populations

    c) Compares breast cancer survival rates in a study population with those expected from cancer registry records of appropriate city, state or nation

    d) Compares breast cancer mortality rates in a study population to those expected from cancer registry records of appropriate city, state or nation

    e) None of the above

6. Concerning minimal breast carcinoma:

    a) It may be defined as all infiltrative cancers less than 1 cm and all in situ cancers

    b) Ten-year survival rates are 95%

    c) Detection rates for minimal breast cancers are 7 times higher in the BCDDP than in the earlier HIP study

    d) 95% of minimal breast cancers at the BCDDP were detected by mammography and 33% by physical examination

    e) All of the above

7. Benefit/risk ratios based on BCDDP data:

    a) Support screening of asymptomatic women only if they are over 50 years of age

    b) Support only a single baseline mammogram for asymptomatic women below age 50

    c) Support annual screening for all asymptomatic women above 35 years of age

    d) All of the above

    e) None of the above

8. Benefit/risk ratios are least necessary in which of the following decisions:

    a) Screening asymptomatic women below 50 years of age

    b) Screening asymptomatic women above 50 years of age

    c) Diagnostic evaluation of women with signs or symptoms of possible breast cancer

    d) Determination of screening frequency

Answers on page 335.

Magnification Mammography: A New Technique for the More Accurate Diagnosis of Breast Cancer

Edward A. Sickles, M.D.

Objectives

1. To describe a new technique for mammography.
2. To present data from a study of use of this new technique vs. conventional mammography.
3. To assess the future role of magnification mammography.

Conventional mammography is currently the most accurate noninvasive means to detect breast cancer, especially the very small tumors that have the greatest potential for cure [1-3]. The radiographic diagnosis of breast cancer rests primarily on the demonstration either of a breast mass having poorly defined stellate margins [4, 5] or of a cluster of tiny rod-shaped calcifications, each calcification no larger than the dots over the i's on this page [6, 7]. Benign breast lesions can also be detected by mammography, characteristically presenting either as masses that have sharply defined margins and smooth contours or as calcifications no larger than their malignant counterparts, but of round or oval shape. To distinguish benign from malignant breast masses requires very fine-detailed images,

Edward A. Sickles, M.D., Chief, Mammography Section, Department of Radiology, University of California School of Medicine, San Francisco.

Based, in part, on a paper with the same title, to be published in *The Female Patient*.

33

to portray the nature of their margins with optimal clarity; equally fine-detailed images are needed to demonstrate the shapes of breast microcalcifications. Lack of sufficient detail, a common problem with conventional mammography techniques, often produces equivocal radiographic interpretations, resulting in biopsy to rule out malignancy. Biopsy of equivocal lesions is widely accepted, and indeed is necessary to detect as many small cancers as possible [4, 5, 7-9]. An unfortunate consequence of this approach, however, is that several benign lesions have to be removed for each malignancy confirmed [10, 11]. The benign/malignant ratio is as high as 10:1 in some centers [9]. By substantially improving the sharpness and detail of the mammographic image, we can expect to convert some of the equivocal mammographic interpretations into definitive diagnoses, either benign or malignant. The technique of direct radiographic magnification offers just this promise, for it has already been documented that the added sharpness of magnification angiographic and skeletal images results in increased diagnostic accuracy for these examinations [12, 13].

Conventional radiographs are taken with the x-ray film in contact with the body part that is being examined, producing an essentially life-sized (contact) image. By increasing the distance between the body part and the film, an enlarged (magnified) x-ray image results. However, magnification radiography will not be successful unless done with a specialized x-ray tube that has an extremely small x-ray source (focal spot), to minimize the blurring that accompanies geometric image enlargement. It has been only within the past five years that such a microfocal spot tube has been constructed to operate at the low x-ray energies required for mammography. Our experience with this equipment* has demonstrated its specific utility in the management of the difficult-to-evaluate equivocal cases that result in so many biopsies for benign lesions.

An initial laboratory evaluation of the microfocal spot mammography apparatus determined the optimal degree of magnification to be 1.5 times life-size [14, 15]. We then began and have since completed a prospective clinical trial to determine the ability of 1.5X magnification imaging to increase

---

*Radiologic Sciences, Inc., a subsidiary of Pfizer, Inc., New York, N.Y.

the accuracy of the conventional mammography examination [16, 17]. Patients were selected for study either because our own conventional mammograms were interpreted as equivocal (suspicious for but not diagnostic of malignancy) or because we knew that breast biopsy was planned in the near future, hence pathologic proof could be expected. Informed consent was obtained for a single additional magnification mammogram and the conventional plus magnification examination was then re-interpreted, by the same observers, who recorded any changes in overall diagnostic impression.

Seven hundred fifty patients were studied, approximately equal numbers with xerographic (blue-and-white) and low-dose film (black-and-white) imaging systems. No differences in results were found between these two imaging systems in any of the subsequent data breakdowns. For almost every patient studied, the single additional 1.5X magnification mammogram presented a sharper, more detailed image of the breast than its conventional (1X) counterparts. Nine breast cancers were detected on the magnification mammogram that had been completely missed on the entire standard examination. Most of these cancers were found by serendipity, since the magnification mammogram was done to evaluate a lesion elsewhere in the breast. The principal impact of magnification mammography, however, was found in the evaluation of lesions interpreted as equivocal on conventional examination. Margins of breast masses and the extent and shapes of clustered breast microcalcifications were often portrayed with so much greater clarity that a definitively benign or malignant diagnosis could be made. Overall, approximately 70% of the cases initially read as equivocal were re-interpreted definitively with the addition of a single magnification mammogram (Table 1). Radiographic-pathologic correlation was done on the 251 patients who underwent biopsy within one month of study. These data, shown in Table 2, indicate the striking increase in diagnostic accuracy of magnification mammography among patients whose conventional mammograms were interpreted as equivocal. Of the 48 cases read as malignant because of the additional magnification mammogram, only one interpretation proved to be in error, and all of the 57 cases read as benign after magnification mammography were indeed benign at biopsy.

Table 1. Diagnostic Interpretations for All 750 Patients Studied

Conventional Mammography	Conventional + Magnification Mammography
227 Benign	201 Benign 19 Equivocal 7 Malignant
496 Equivocal	297 Benign 151 Equivocal 48 Malignant
27 Malignant	27 Malignant

The increased diagnostic accuracy of magnification mammography translates readily into improved patient management. Magnification mammography has caused many cancers to be removed more promptly than would have been done otherwise, either because it detected malignant lesions that were not even suspected on conventional mammograms or because it definitively demonstrated malignancy in lesions that were judged to be only equivocal by conventional mammography. (Despite our suggestion to biopsy equivocal lesions, occasionally the surgeon or the patient elects to defer biopsy in favor of clinical observation.) However, the most dramatic effect of magnification mammography on patient management has been a substantial reduction in the number of biopsies for benign lesions,

Table 2. Diagnostic Interpretations with Pathological Correlation
for the 251 Biopsy-Proved Cases

Mammographic Diagnosis		Pathological Diagnosis
Conventional	Conventional + Magnification	
56 Benign	38 Benign 12 Equivocal 6 Malignant	36 Benign, 2 malignant 9 Benign, 3 malignant 6 Malignant
168 Equivocal	57 Benign 63 Equivocal 48 Malignant	57 Benign 44 Benign, 19 malignant 1 Benign, 47 malignant
27 Malignant	27 Malignant	27 Malignant

i.e. cases in which the magnification mammogram eliminated the suspicion of malignancy that had been indicated by the conventional examination. Although there is no histological proof in these cases, we are now following almost 250 such women, some for as long as 4½ years, and none has developed cancer in or adjacent to the area where conventional mammograms initially suggested some suspicion of malignancy.

The precise role of magnification mammography has not yet been established, but it certainly appears to be of value as an adjunct to conventional mammography when the initial study is read as equivocal for malignancy. We do not, however, recommend magnification examinations in place of conventional mammography, primarily because we would expect a much lower number of changed diagnoses in a consecutive series of unselected patients than the dramatic increase in accuracy observed in our study of difficult-to-evaluate patients. A secondary but quite valid concern is that magnification mammography results in radiation doses to the breast 1½ to 4 times higher than standard contact mammography [14, 16]. Each magnification exposure produces a breast tissue dose of ½ to ¼ rad, a dose that is totally acceptable for the one-time evaluation of a radiographically suspicious lesion, for which the likelihood of malignancy is relatively high. On the other hand, a complete examination with the magnification technique would require at least two exposures per breast; if repeated examinations are planned for an asymptomatic patient population (very low yield of breast cancer), lower dose contact mammography seems a more prudent alternative, at least for the present time. This may well change, however, because magnification mammography is also quite feasible using ultrafast screen-film systems, producing substantially reduced radiation doses [16, 18, 19]. We are, in fact, currently evaluating several such systems to determine whether the improved diagnostic accuracy of magnification mammography is also observed at radiation doses equal to and lower than those of conventional contact examinations.

The last and ultimate factors in determining what role magnification mammography will play in the detection of breast cancer are the twin considerations of availability and cost. As discussed previously, magnification mammography cannot be done with conventional x-ray equipment; it requires a microfocal spot x-ray tube specially adapted for mammography. In major medical centers and also in many private radiology offices, mammography is already done with specialized x-ray units dedicated specifically to mammographic use. As this equipment wears out or otherwise becomes obsolete, replacement with a microfocal spot unit rather than with a larger focal spot model should not involve any extra cost, since microfocal spot systems do both contact and magnification mammography and since they are currently sold at the competitive price of approximately $49,000. However, an expenditure of this magnitude to replace existing equipment that is in good working order, especially if it is of the cheaper, nondedicated (general-purpose) type, will certainly result in some cost increase. Considered in the context of the current lay-press "radiation scare," with the resultant (inappropriate and unfortunate) nationwide decline in mammography utilization, economic considerations have, in most instances, been the primary reasons for radiologists to continue with the poorer image quality, less accurate mammography units they already have. At present, 25 microfocal spot mammography units are in operation in the United States, mostly in hospitals but also in some private radiology offices. In time, more and more radiologists will replace worn-out mammography equipment with microfocal spot systems, because they produce superior-quality images at equal cost. On the other hand, there probably will not be a widespread scrapping of well-functioning conventional units unless sufficient demand comes from referring physicians.

Summary

A new x-ray unit designed specifically for mammography produces magnified images of the breast that are sharper and more detailed than conventional mammograms. A prospective clinical trial involving 750 patients has demonstrated that the additional diagnostic information provided in magnification mammograms can substantially increase the accuracy of radiographic interpretation. In some cases, breast cancer completely missed by conventional mammography was detected on a single additional magnification image. Of much greater impact, however, was the ability of magnification mammography to definitively indicate malignancy or benignity among patients whose conventional mammograms were given equivocal interpretations. The net result was more prompt biopsy of some breast cancers and a substantial reduction in the number of biopsies for benign lesions.

References

1. Feig, S.A., Shaber, G.S., Schwartz, G.F. et al: Thermography, mammography, and clinical examination in breast cancer screening. Review of 16,000 studies. Radiology 122:123-127, Jan. 1977.
2. Feig, S.A., Shaber, G.S., Patchefsky, A. et al: Analysis of clinically occult and mammographically occult breast tumors. AJR 128:403-408, Mar. 1977.
3. Feig, S.A., Schwartz, G.F., Nerlinger, R. et al: Prognostic factors of breast neoplasms detected on screening by mammography and physical examination. Radiology 133:577-582, Dec. 1979.
4. Wolfe, J.N.: Xeroradiography: Uncalcified Breast Masses. Springfield: Charles C Thomas, 1977, pp. 3-41.
5. Martin, J.E.: Correlations of mammography and histology of the breast, benign and malignant. In Margulis, A.R. and Gooding, C.A. (eds.): Diagnostic Radiology 1977. San Francisco:University of California Press, 1977, pp. 807-821.
6. Martin, J.E.: Benign vs. malignant calcifications. In Margulis, A.R. and Gooding, C.A. (eds.): Diagnostic Radiology 1977. San Francisco: University of California Press, 1977, pp. 831-836.
7. Wolfe, J.N.: Xeroradiography: Breast Calcifications. Springfield: Charles C Thomas, 1977, pp. 3-43.
8. Gold, R.H.: Breast. In Steckel, R.J. and Kagan, A.R. (eds.): Diagnosis and Staging of Cancer. A Radiologic Approach. Philadelphia:W. B. Saunders, 1976, pp. 263-287.
9. Moskowitz, M., Gartside, P.S., Gardella, L. et al: The breast cancer screening controversy: A perspective. In Logan, W.W. (ed.): Breast Carcinoma. The Radiologist's Expanded Role. New York:John Wiley & Sons, 1977, pp. 35-52.
10. Rosen, P.P. and Snyder, R.E.: Nonpalpable breast lesions detected by mammography and confirmed by specimen radiography — Recent experience. Breast 3:13-16, April-July 1977.
11. Cheek, J.H.: Experience with breast biopsies for mammographic findings. Breast 4:4-9, Jan.-March 1978.
12. Takahashi, S., Sakuma, S., Kaneko, M. et al: Angiography at fourfold magnification with special reference to the examination of tumours. Acta Radiol. (Diag.) 4:206-216, March 1966.
13. Genant, H.K., Doi, K., Mall, J.C. et al: Direct radiographic magnification for skeletal radiology. An assessment of image quality and clinical application. Radiology 123:47-55, April 1977.
14. Sickles, E.A., Doi, K. and Genant, H.K.: Magnification film mammography: Image quality and clinical studies. Radiology 125:69-76, Oct. 1977.

15. Nguyen, M.T. and Sickles, E.A.: Radiographic detectability of breast microcalcifications: *in vitro* studies using a wide variety of mammography techniques. *In* Application of Optical Instrumentation in Medicine VII. Bellingham, Wash.:Society of Photo-Optical Instrumentation Engineers, 1979, pp. 129-134.
16. Sickles, E.A.: Microfocal spot magnification mammography using xeroradiographic and screen-film recording systems. Radiology 131:599-607, June 1979.
17. Sickles, E.A.: Further experience with microfocal spot magnification mammography in the assessment of clustered breast microcalcifications. Radiology. (In press.)
18. Arnold, B.A., Eisenberg, H. and Bjarngard, B.: Low-dose magnification mammography. Radiology 131:743-749, June 1979.
19. Kubo, K.: Recent development of magnification technique in mammography and its diagnostic significance. Presented at XII International Cancer Congress, Buenos Aires, Oct. 5-11, 1978.

Self-Evaluation Quiz

1. Characteristic mammographic features of breast cancer include:
   a) At least ten microcalcifications within a 1-mm^3 volume
   b) Clustered rod-shaped microcalcifications
   c) Clustered round microcalcifications
   d) Microcalcifications scattered throughout the breast
2. Characteristic mammographic features of breast cancer include:
   a) Poorly defined mass with spiculated margins
   b) Sharply defined mass with gently lobulated contour
   c) Sharply defined mass with smooth, round contour
   d) Breast mass larger than 2.5 cm
3. Most breast biopsies generated solely by abnormal mammography examinations show benign rather than malignant histology.
   a) True
   b) False
4. The statement in question #3 is best explained by:
   a) The relatively high diagnostic accuracy of breast cancer detection by mammography
   b) The relatively low diagnostic accuracy of breast cancer detection by physical examination
   c) The frequent inability of mammography to diagnose nonpalpable benign breast lesions as being unequivocally benign

    d) The frequent inability of mammography to diagnose nonpalpable breast cancers as being unequivocally malignant

5. Magnification mammography can be done successfully using:
    a) Conventional xeromammography equipment, with minor modifications in radiographic technique
    b) Conventional low-dose film mammography equipment, with minor modifications in radiographic technique
    c) Conventional xeromammography or low-dose film mammography equipment, but only after considerable alteration in radiographic technique and patient positioning technique
    d) A specialized x-ray tube that has an extremely small focal spot

6. Advantages of magnification mammography include:
    a) Increased image detail
    b) Larger image size
    c) Increased diagnostic accuracy
    d) All of the above

7. Major reasons for the improved results achieved by magnification mammography include:
    a) Ability to more accurately determine number of breast microcalcifications
    b) Ability to more accurately determine size of breast masses
    c) Superior ability to portray shapes of microcalcifications and margins of masses
    d) All of the above

8. The major impact of magnification mammography on patient management has been:
    a) Reduction in the number of breast biopsies
    b) Reduction in the number of biopsies of benign breast lesions
    c) Increase in the number of biopsies of malignant breast lesions
    d) Earlier detection of breast cancer

9. Magnification mammography currently should be used:
    a) For all women undergoing mammography
    b) Only for women over the age of 50

    c) Only for women at high risk for developing breast cancer

    d) Only for women in whom conventional mammography produces equivocal results

10. Current obstacles to the widespread acceptance of magnification mammography include:

    a) Lack of awareness by referring physicians of its potential benefits

    b) Limited availability of appropriate x-ray equipment

    c) Higher radiation dose than conventional mammography

    d) All of the above

Answers on page 335.

Computed Tomographic Evaluation of Breast Cancer

C. H. Joseph Chang, M.D.

Objectives

1. To report our experiences with computed tomographic mammography (CT/M) in the diagnosis of breast cancers.
2. To compare the results with film mammography, breast thermography and physical examination for histologically proven cases of mammary cancer.
3. To present our experiences with CT/M as a risk indicator for potentially precancerous breast lesions.

Elevated iodine and iodide concentrations in breast carcinoma have been well documented [1-4]. However, this metabolic abnormality has never become a clinical method of detecting breast cancer because of inadequate detector systems.

The General Electric Computed Tomographic Breast Scanner (CT/M) is a dedicated breast scanner. A CT/M study using our contrast medium enhancement technique can not only identify static anatomical changes in the breast but can measure abnormal iodide concentrations in mammary tissues. This unique capability of CT/M provides many advantages, as compared with conventional mammography.

During the period from October 1, 1976 to January 3, 1980, we evaluated 1,846 patients with the CT/M system at our institution. The purpose of this paper is to report our experiences with CT/M in the diagnosis of breast cancers. The results are compared with film mammography, breast thermography and physical examination for histologically proven cases

C. H. Joseph Chang, M.D., Department of Diagnostic Radiology, Kansas University Medical Center, Kansas City, Kan.

of mammary cancer. Our experiences with CT/M as a risk indicator for precancerous breast lesions will also be presented.

The General Electric CT/M System

The GE CT/M system is a prototype CT fan-beam scanner that is specially designed for breast scanning. The system includes a three-phase x-ray generator, GE Maxiray 75 tube, an array of 127 high-pressure xenon gas detectors, Data General S/200 Eclipse Computer with magnetic tape drive, Control Data Corp. (CDC) disc, RAMTEC display console, Versatec printer and Dunn camera. The scanning field is 20 cm in diameter. The resolution volume for each picture point is $1.56 \times 1.56 \times 10.00$ mm. Reconstruction requires 90 seconds per slide. Images from the 127×127 matrix are displayed on a scale of -127 to $+127$ CT numbers with water calibrated at zero.

The scanning is done at 120 KVp, 20 ma (HVL $-$ 3.4 mm Al). A 1-cm slice of the breast is scanned in 10 seconds. The average midbreast radiation dose for a six-slice examination has been measured to be 0.175 rad. This is much less than the single-view, average midbreast dose of 0.370 rad using xero-mammography for the same size breast [5] and more than a single-view, low-dose film mammography examination of 0.04 rad [5].

Materials and Methods

A total of 1,846 patients was studied with the CT/M system from October 1, 1976 through January 3, 1980. All underwent physical examination, low-dose film mammography and breast thermography. Six groups of patients were selected for this study: (1) patients with physical, mammographic and/or major thermographic abnormalities; (2) asymptomatic patients in a high-risk group; (3) asymptomatic patients with dysplastic dense breasts; (4) post-cobalt therapy patients; (5) post-lumpectomy and chemotherapy patients; and (6) patients with silicone mammoplasty. The majority of patients, however, are from groups 2 and 3.

The patient stands on a platform with her body flat against the canvas table in slight obliquity so that her breast can project through the center of the opening. After being stabilized, she is gently lowered to the horizontal position until the breast is completely immersed in the water container. Horizontal scans are obtained from the chest wall to the nipple. The required CT slices can be predetermined by looking at the breast through a mirror system. CT scans are obtained before and after the rapid intravenous drip infusion of 300 ml of diatrizoate meglumine.*

For every lesion, the highest CT value has been utilized instead of average CT number values. The final CT values were obtained on hard-copy print. All lesions were localized by fixing the position of the lesion in relation to the nipple. The nipple was marked by superimposing a slice containing a nipple shadow. Localization of a lesion was described in a clockwise direction and distance was directly measured from the nipple. The depth of a lesion was obtained by subtracting the scan slice containing the lesion from the scan containing the nipple shadow. Since there is no compression of the breast during an examination, CT/M is more accurate than film mammographic localization.

CT/M Findings in Breast Cancers

From the 1,846 patients studied, 92 histologically proven carcinomas and one cystosarcoma phyllodes have been detected in 86 patients. The histological details of the 93 malignancies are described in Table 1. The size of cancers has ranged from 2 mm to 9 cm in maximum diameter. Twenty-seven were less than 1 cm in diameter, 29 were 1 to 2 cm, 18 were 2 to 3 cm, 10 were 3 to 5 cm, and 8 were over 5 cm. The cystosarcoma phyllodes measured 3.5 cm.

Breast cancer in fatty breasts is characterized on a CT/M scan as an irregular mass which exhibits markedly increased CT numbers on the postinjection scan. In moderate to markedly dense fibrocystic breasts, and occasionally even with minimal disease, a cancer can be obscured by surrounding mammary tissues on mammograms. In these latter cases, the precontrast CT/M scan failed to distinguish a tumor mass from surrounding tissue. The cancer becomes obvious on a postinjection scan because of preferential high iodide uptake by the tumor. Malignant microcalcifications without an associated mass cannot be identified on a preinjection scan because of the averaging

---

*Reno-M-30-DIP, E. R. Squibb & Sons, Inc., Princeton, New Jersey.

Table 1. Histological Classification of 93 Malignancies

Ductal carcinoma	
Invasive, type unspecified	59
Scirrhous type	3
Medullary type	4
Comedo type	3
Papillary type	2
Tubular type	1
Mucinous (colloid) type	2
Adenoid cystic type	1
In situ	1
	76
Lobular carcinoma	
Invasive	11
In situ	4
	15
Mixed invasive ductal and lobular carcinoma	1
Malignant cystosarcoma phyllodes	1

effect within the computer matrix, but they can be shown as tiny areas of marked contrast enhancement on postinjection scans. Biopsy-proven recurrent cancer in two post-cobalt therapy patients with advanced cancer also showed high contrast enhancement. A patient with benign postirradiation fibrosis, however, failed to show any significant contrast enhancement.

A small cancer in the wall of a benign cyst is one of the hardest diagnoses for mammography or physical examination to make. CT/M, however, detected a small cancer by identifying high concentration of iodide in the wall of the cyst. Another exciting contribution of CT/M is the detection of totally occult microcarcinomas, even in fatty breasts.

The CT/M is able to differentiate, preoperatively, benign skin thickening from cutaneous invasion from breast cancer by identifying high contrast-medium enhancement of over 25 CT numbers (50 Hounsfield units). Benign skin thickening shows less than 10 CT number enhancement on the postcontrast scan.

The initial CT number of breast cancers ranged from -19 (-38 Hounsfield units) to 39 (78 Hounsfield units) (mean 19, or 38 Hounsfield units), and $+10 \sim +96$ ($20 \sim 192$ Hounsfield units) (mean 53, or 106 Hounsfield units) on postinjection contrast media scans. The mean CT number increase from precontrast scan to postcontrast scan (ΔCT number) in proven breast cancers was 34 (68 Hounsfield units). Eighty-one cancers showed an increase of at least 26 CT numbers (52 Hounsfield units) after contrast medium enhancement. Five cancers exhibited an increase of 20 (40 Hounsfield units) to 23 CT numbers (46 Hounsfield units). Three cancers showed 18 (36 Hounsfield units), 13 (26 Hounsfield units), and 11 CT number (22 Hounsfield units) enhancement, respectively. One cancer failed to show any significant contrast enhancement. Preinjection CT number for the malignant cystosarcoma phyllodes was 19 (38 Hounsfield units) and 62 (124 Hounsfield units) on the postcontrast scan, which showed ΔCT number of 43 (86 Hounsfield units).

The detection rate of CT/M for the 92 cancers and one cystosarcoma phyllodes, compared to those for low-dose film mammography, thermography and physical examination, is summarized in Table 2. Eighty-seven of 93 malignancies (94%) were diagnosed by CT/M study, while only 72 malignancies (77%) were detected by mammography. Mammography missed 11 cancers in dense fibrocystic breasts and 2 recurrent cancers in post-cobalt therapy breasts with marked fibrosis. All 93 malignancies were detected by using both CT/M and mammography. The detection rate for breast thermography was 53% and 62% for physical examination.

The greatest value of CT/M is the detection of cancer in dense, premenopausal dysplastic breasts (DY). Mammography is of very limited value in this patient group due to a lack of tissue contrast. There were 14 cancers in DY breasts; mammography detected only 3 of these (21%), but CT/M correctly diagnosed all 14 (100%).

Table 2. Comparative Diagnostic Accuracy
in 93 Malignant Lesions

	Not Detected	Benign	Suspicious	Malignant
Film mammography	5	16	36	36 (77%)
Thermography	44	–	21	28 (53%)
Physical examination	11	24	48	10 (62%)
CT/M	2	4	5	82 (94%)
Mammography + CT/M	–	–	6	87 (100%)

CT/M as a Risk Indicator for Potentially
Precancerous Breast Lesions

Breast cancer may develop more often when epithelial proliferative disorders, such as atypical terminal duct epithelial hyperplasia and atypical lobular hyperplasia, are present [4, 6-15]. A fivefold increased risk of developing breast cancer in women with this condition was reported by Black and his co-workers [6]. Recently Page et al [13] reported a six-times elevated risk factor for women under 45 years with atypical lobular hyperplasia and tripling of the risk factor in the patient population after the age of 45 years. They also reported a doubly increased risk with various ductal hyperplastic lesions when the lesions are identified at biopsy after the age of 45 years. Moskowitz et al [4] described a 13-times greater risk for women with atypical hyperplasia.

Abnormal xeromammographic patterns [16] and microcalcifications [17] have been used to predict the risk of developing breast cancer. Wellings and Wolfe [18] reported the highest grade of precancerous epithelial abnormality found in P2 and DY breasts. However, other investigators [19-23] either refute or incompletely support the concept of mammographic patterns as risk markers. Abnormal breast patterns, even DY breasts, cannot always indicate the presence of epithelial hyperplasia. The mammographic changes are often due to marked fibrosis, which is not considered to be a precancerous lesion. Microcalcifications may be related to previous disease and do not specify present active pathology or identify the exact location of abnormal cellular activity.

The preoperative diagnosis of potentially precancerous breast lesions by CT/M was initially reported by our group [7]. We have now detected 71 areas of terminal duct epithelial hyperplasia, with various degrees of cellular atypia, in 60 patients. All lesions were biopsied solely on the basis of the CT/M abnormalities. The CT/M scan characteristically showed two or three tiny areas, often bilateral, of increased contrast enhancement, above 25 CT numbers (50 Hounsfield units).

Our initial data indicate that CT/M has the ability to differentiate potentially precancerous epithelial proliferative lesions from non-precancerous bland fibrocystic diseases, by identifying tiny areas of increased iodide uptake. The latter condition exhibits no significant contrast enhancement (usually less than 10 CT numbers).

Discussion

Our results confirm the previously reported findings of increased iodide uptake in breast cancer [1, 2, 24, 25]. The CT/M system provides a new method of detecting breast cancers, utilizing dynamic measurement of abnormal iodide concentration. In the diagnosis of breast carcinoma, CT/M appears to be superior to all other modalities. It also appears to be a potential risk indicator for precancerous lesions.

A lesion with contrast medium enhancement (ΔCT number of over 25 CT numbers) strongly supports the diagnosis of malignancy and a contrast enhancement above 20 CT numbers is suspicious for cancer. Contrast enhancement above 25 CT numbers has also been found in noncalcified fibroadenomas, breast abscesses, comedomastitis, angiolipoma, hyperprolactinemia and an infected cyst. However, the precontrast mean CT number for fibroadenoma is only 12 (24 Hounsfield units) and for abscesses 17 (34 Hounsfield units). It is 19 (38 Hounsfield units) for breast cancers. Roentgenographically, a fibroadenoma appears as a well-defined, smooth, homogenous, oval mass, as do angiolipomas. Abscesses have usually been located close to the skin. Infected cysts show a characteristically increased iodide uptake around the rim of the cyst. Comedomastitis, however, can mimic a cancer, and it can be the cause of a false-positive finding.

Minimal contrast enhancement, less than 10 CT numbers (20 Hounsfield units), characterized benign fibrotic and cystic lesions of the breast. In 129 histologically proven benign lesions, 35 cases (27%) — including 23 fibrocystic diseases, 4 abscesses and 8 comedomastitis — mimicked malignancies by CT/M study, while 55 cases (43%) were incorrectly diagnosed as cancers by mammography.

Our clinical experiences indicate that there is a definite relationship between iodide concentration in mammary tissue and a high level of progesterone and prolactin. Eskin reported two- to five-fold increased uptake of radioactive iodine in rat breasts with estrogen and two- to four-fold increased uptake with testosterone [3]. Estrogen and other hormones may also

VANDERBILT MEDICAL CENTER LIBRARY

affect the iodide concentration in the human breast tissue. CT/M scan findings reflecting these abnormal hormonal effects usually showed multiple, tiny areas of marked contrast enhancement, over 25 CT numbers (50 Hounsfield units) throughout both breasts. These are distinguished easily from cancer.

Other significant contributions of CT/M have been the detection of totally occult microcarcinomas, the preoperative diagnosis of a tiny cancer in the wall of a benign cyst and the prebiopsy identification of potentially precancerous lesions. This hopefully will bring a significant improvement to both early detection and the survival rate of breast cancer. Since CT/M is now able to detect very small cancers and precancerous lesions, extraordinary cooperation between the surgeon and pathologist is required to find these lesions in the specimen.

The need for intravenous infusion of iodinated contrast medium with the CT/M study has been well established [1, 2, 7]. Of the 1,846 patients scanned with the use of contrast material, 73 patients (4%) experienced minor reactions, primarily hives and itching; only 8 patients (0.43%) had moderate reactions. These are well within the reported incidence of such reactions [26]. There was no fatal reaction in our series.

Currently, the General Electric Company has decided not to market the CT/M scanner. The CT/M prototype scanner at the Mayo Clinic was removed from service in August 1979. The CT/M prototype scanner at the University of Kansas Medical Center was removed in January 1980. At the present time, we are working on a technique to study breasts using a conventional CT body scanner. Our preliminary experience in the diagnosis of breast cancer using the GE body scanner (CT/T 8800 unit) is encouraging.

Summary

From October 1, 1976 through January 3, 1980, 1,846 patients were examined by CT/M at the University of Kansas Medical Center. Ninety-two cancers and one cystosarcoma phyllodes were histologically diagnosed.

The unique capability of CT/M for detecting both anatomical changes and abnormal iodide concentrations in breast cancer provides many advantages over conventional mammography in the diagnosis of mammary cancer. The detection rate in 93 malignancies by CT/M was 94% vs. 77% for mammography.

CT/M appears to be especially superior to mammography for detecting cancers in dense, premenopausal dysplastic breasts. The CT/M can detect totally unsuspected, very small cancers which are occult by conventional mammography or physical examination. A CT/M scan may also be a valid test for recognizing precancerous high-risk lesions. This will hopefully bring a significant improvement to both early detection and the survival rate of breast cancer.

The need for intravenous infusion of contrast medium, high cost of the examination and lengthy procedure make CT/M inappropriate as a screening tool for the general population. The CT/M examination, however, affords definitive diagnosic help in an instance where the mammographic and/or physical examinations are inconclusive. Although CT/M will not replace conventional mammography in routine breast examinations, it overcomes many limitations of mammography. CT/M appears to be a significantly improved new method of breast cancer diagnosis.

References

1. Chang, C.H.J., Sibala, J.L., Gallagher, J.H. et al: Computed tomography of the breast: A preliminary report. Radiology 124:827-829, 1977.
2. Chang, C.H.J., Sibala, J.L., Fritz, S.L. et al: Computed tomographic evaluation of the breast. AJR 131:459-464, 1978.
3. Eskin, B.A.: Iodine metabolism and breast cancer. Trans. N.Y. Acad. Sci. 32:911-947, 1970.
4. Moskowitz, M., Gartside, P., Wirman, J.A. and McLaughlin, C.: Proliferative disorders of the breast as risk factors for breast cancer in a self-selected screened population: Pathologic markers. Radiology 134:289-291, 1980.
5. Hammerstein, G.R., Miller, D.W., White, D.R. et al: Absorbed radiation dose in mammography. Radiology 130:485-491, 1979.
6. Black, M.M., Barclay, T.H., Cutler, S.J. et al: Association of atypical characteristics of benign breast lesions with subsequent risk of breast cancer. Cancer 29:339-343, 1972.
7. Chang, C.H.J., Sibala, J.L., Lin, F. et al: Preoperative diagnosis of potentially precancerous breast lesions by computed tomographic breast scanner: Preliminary study. Radiology 129:209-210, 1978.
8. Dawson, E.K.: Carcinoma in mammary lobule and its origin. Edinburgh Med. J. 40:57-82, 1933.
9. Foote, F.W. and Stewart, F.W.: Comparative studies of cancerous versus noncancerous breasts. Ann. Surg. 121:6-53, 1945.

10. Humphrey, L.J. and Swerdlow, M.: Relationship of benign breast disease to carcinoma of the breast. Surgery 52:841-846, 1962.
11. Kern, W.H. and Brooks, R.N.: Atypical epithelial hyperplasia associated with breast cancer and fibrocystic disease. Cancer 24:668-675, 1969.
12. Muir, R.: The evaluation of carcinoma of the mamma. J. Pathol. Bacteriol. 52:155-172, 1941.
13. Page, D.L., Zwaag, R.V., Rogers, L.W. et al: Relation between component parts of fibrocystic disease complex and breast cancer. JNCI 61:1055-1063, 1978.
14. Ryan, J.A. and Coady, C.J.: Ductal proliferation in breast cancer. Can. J. Surg. 5:12-19, 1952.
15. Wellings, S.R. and Jensen, H.M.: An atlas of subgross pathology of the human breast with special reference to possible precancerous lesions. JNCI 55:231-273, 1975.
16. Wolfe, J.N.: Breast patterns as an index of risk for developing breast cancer. AJR 226:1130-1139, 1976.
17. Price, J.L. and Gibbs, N.M.: The relationships between microcalcification and in situ carcinoma of the breast. Clin. Radiol. 29:447-452, 1978.
18. Wellings, S.R. and Wolfe, J.N.: Correlation studies of the histological and radiographic appearance of the breast parenchyma. Radiology 129:299-306, 1978.
19. Eagon, R.L. and Mosteller, R.C.: Breast cancer mammography patterns. Cancer 40:2087-2090, 1977.
20. Mendell, L., Rosenbloom, M. and Naimark, A.: Are breast patterns a risk for breast cancer? A reappraisal. AJR 128:547, 1977.
21. Moskowitz, M., Gartside, P. and McLaughlin, C.: Mammographic patterns as markers for high-risk benign breast disease and incident cancers. Radiology 134:293-295, 1980.
22. Peyster, R.G., Kalisher, L. and Cole, P.: Mammographic parenchymal patterns and the prevalence of breast cancer. Radiology 125:387-391, 1977.
23. Rideout, D.F. and Poon, P.Y.: Patterns of breast parenchyma on mammography. J. Can. Assoc. Radiol. 28:257-258, 1977.
24. Eskin, B.A., Parker, J.A., Bassett, J.G. and George, D.L.: Human breast uptake of radioactive iodine. Obstet. Gynecol. 44:398-402, 1974.
25. Palmer, R.C.: Final Report GM 15814. Radionuclide-labeled compound for tumor localization. April 1969 - December 1972. (Unpublished.)
26. Witten, D.M., Hirsch, F.D. and Hartman, G.W.: Acute reactions to urographic contrast medium. AJR 119:832-840, 1973.

Self-Evaluation Quiz

1. Iodide concentration in breast cancer is:
   a) Unchanged

   b) Elevated

   c) Decreased

2. Computed tomographic mammography (CT/M) using contrast medium enhancement technique can identify:

   a) Anatomical changes in the breast

   b) Abnormal iodide concentrations in the breast

   c) All of the above

Match the following average midbreast radiation dose for a 6-cm breast with the correct technique:

____ 3. Xeromammography   a) 0.04 rad

____ 4. CT/M   b) 0.37 rad

____ 5. Low-dose film mammography   c) 0.175 rad

6. The film mammographic localization of breast lesions is more accurate than CT/M localization.

   a) True

   b) False

7. Breast cancer in a fatty breast is characterized on CT/M scan as:

   a) Irregular mass

   b) Smooth mass

   c) Microcalcification

   d) Irregular mass and markedly increased CT numbers on the postcontrast scan

   e) High initial CT values

8. Malignant microcalcification without an associated mass can be identified on a preinjection CT/M scan.

   a) True

   b) False

9. CT/M study can detect mammographically and physically occult microcarcinomas.

   a) True

   b) False

10. The breast carcinomas will exhibit contrast medium enhancement (CT number) of:

   a) 10 CT numbers (20 Hounsfield units)

   b) 15 CT numbers (30 Hounsfield units)

   c) Over 25 CT numbers (50 Hounsfield units)

   d) 0 CT numbers

   e) 5 CT numbers (10 Hounsfield units)

11. The diagnostic accuracy of CT/M study in 93 malignant
    lesions was:
    a) 62%
    b) 77%
    c) 94%
    d) 53%
12. The CT/M appears to be especially superior to mammog-
    raphy for detecting breast cancers in:
    a) Fatty breasts
    b) Large breasts
    c) Small breasts
    d) Dense dysplastic breasts
    e) All of the above
13. A CT/M scan may be a valid test for recognizing precan-
    cerous, high-risk breast lesions.
    a) True
    b) False
14. Contrast medium enhancement above 25 CT numbers has
    been found in:
    a) Breast cancer
    b) Noncalcified fibroadenoma
    c) Breast abscess
    d) Angiolipoma
    e) Hyperprolactinemia
    f) All of the above
15. The CT/M is an ideal screening tool for the general
    population.
    a) True
    b) False

Answers on page 335.

So-Called Mammographic Risk Patterns

Robert L. Egan, M.D.

Objectives

One radiologist claims that women with radiographically dense breasts have such a high risk of cancer that prophylactic mastectomies should be strongly advised. Since this cannot be substantiated and women, especially the younger who normally have dense breast tissues, are being frightened, contrary established facts need to be set forth:

1. Most breast cancers occur in older women with less dense breasts.
2. Cancers in dense breasts are more difficult to detect by mammography and tend to remain prevalent.
3. Radiographic parenchymal patterns cannot be used to select asymptomatic women at a high risk or a low risk.

Complex factors, endocrine, genetic, environmental and behavioral, have been observed in relation to breast cancer. No single epidemiologic, clinical, histopathologic, radiographic or laboratory marker has been capable of placing women at a significant risk for breast cancer. Kelsey's extensive epidemiologic review [1] indicates increasing age, history of bilateral premenopausal breast cancer in a first-degree relative, a history of breast cancer in the contralateral breast and long residence in North America are associated with increased relative risks of breast cancer. Most clinical signs indicate advanced cancer, except a few such as nipple changes of Paget disease or bloody nipple discharge. Radiographic detail of clinical mammog-

Robert L. Egan, M.D., Chief, Mammography Section; Professor of Radiology, Emory University, Atlanta, Ga.

raphy [2] signaled the potential extension of efforts to associate risk with histologic patterns of the breast [3, 4]. Prebiopsy mammograms with histopathologic correlation confirmed a close association of ductal epithelial hyperplasia with breast cancer [5, 6].

Wolfe reported in a retrospective study, based on four levels of increasing amounts and density of breast tissues by x-ray, that, during a 2½ year follow-up period, 22 times as many cancers developed six months or longer after normal mammograms in densest, most glandular breasts as in least dense fatty breasts [7]. On the basis of this observation many women are being told that they have dense fibroglandular breasts by x-ray and have such a high risk of breast cancer that prophylactic mastectomies are strongly advised. Most younger women have radiographically dense breasts.

The Emory University prospective series of x-ray breast cancer risk analysis, of considerable length and size and with adequate follow-up, had failed to demonstrate any significant parenchymal risk pattern other than ductal hyperplasia. It seemed relevant to reexamine our data.

Materials and Methods

At Emory University Clinic from 1963 through 1977, 864 operable primary breast cancers were demonstrated following 1 to 11 clinical and x-ray examinations of the breasts in 7,123 women over 30 years of age. The women were referred from the oncologic clinic for specific breast complaints, for reevaluation of previous breast complaints or as part of a medical examination. The patients were in the upper socioeconomic levels and provided good follow-up. In 82.2% of the cancers, the axillary lymph nodes were free from metastases; 18.2% of the cancers were in clinically normal breasts.

There were 658 prevalent operable primary cancers, defined as those diagnosed within six months of the initial radiographic studies, and 206 incident cancers, those diagnosed at least six months after noncancer clinical and radiographic studies.

A description of the relative amounts, arrangements and location of the fat and fibroglandular tissues and the radiographic appearance of all the women's breasts had been prospectively recorded without knowledge of the individual patient's history or clinical findings [8, 9]. Parenchymal patterns of the breasts were classified into four basic categories previously described [7] as possible risk indicators for breast cancer: N1 as most fatty (Fig. 1), P1 with up to one fourth of the breast containing fibroglandular tissue (Fig. 2), P2 with fibroglandular tissue throughout the breast (Fig. 3), and DY with dense tissues that obscure any underlying fibroglandular tissue (Fig. 4). Extensive testing of pattern recognition by two radiologists for inter- and intra-observer performance was highly consistent using this classification.

Most women developing cancer returned for follow-up. The mammography files, the clinic and hospital charts and the Emory tumor registry were searched for additional women developing breast cancers. Other sources included physicians' personal records at Emory University Clinic, the Georgia Department of Human Resources and printout listings for each of the last three years by the Atlanta SEER Program (Surveillance, Epidemiology and End Results).

Results

There were more glandular breasts (P2, DY) in the younger women and more fatty and less dense breasts (N1, P1) in the older women. One third of the total cancers and one third of the incident (developing) cancers occurred before age 50 years. The average time from the latest noncancer mammogram was 40 months for N1, P1 and 30 months for P2, DY.

The N1, P1 patterns occurred in fewer women but were associated with a higher rate of breast cancer (Table 1). There were three times as many incident cancers in P2, DY as in N1, P1.

The rates of total cancers in most age groups in both N1, P1 and P2, DY were similar (Table 2). Yet, in these same age groups there were 12 times as many incident cancers in P2, DY as in N1, P1 by age 54.

The histopathologic stage of cancer varied little though there were 12 lobular carcinomas in situ in DY and 6 lobular carcinomas in situ in P2 (Table 3). The mortality from breast cancers in DY pattern was 170% of the mortality from cancers in N1 pattern (Table 4).

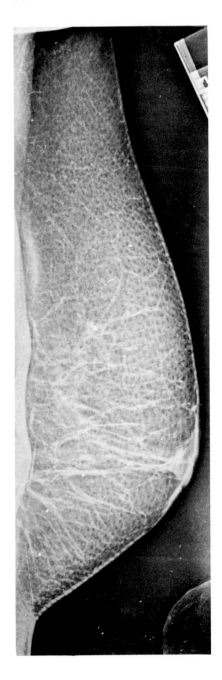

FIG. 1. N1 pattern. The parenchyma is primarily fat without
fibroglandular tissue.

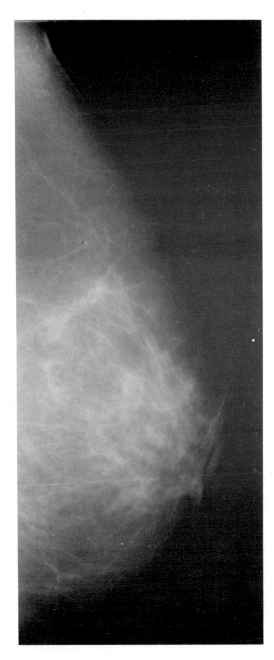

FIG. 2. P1 pattern. Same as N1 except up to one quarter of the breast contains fibro-glandular tissue.

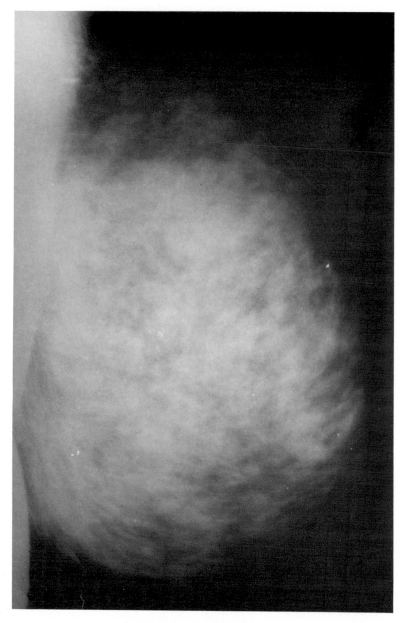

FIG. 3. P2 pattern. Fibroglandular tissue throughout the breast.

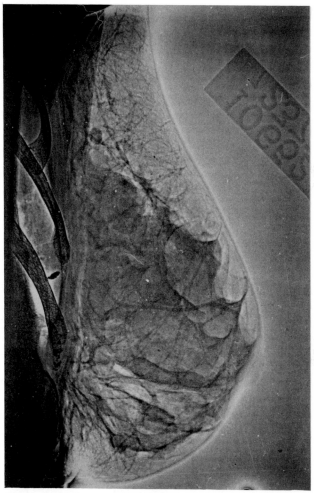

FIG. 4. DY pattern. Severe involvement with dysplastic tissue that often obscures underlying fibroglandular tissue.

Discussion

The sharp reduction in women (derived from Table 2) with P2, DY patterns from 1,104 women aged 30 to 34 years to 264 women over age 70 years (compared with N1, P1 — 667 aged 30 to 34 and 506 over age 70) and increasing rates of cancers with aging suggest that there is within this large group of P2, DY a limited subset of women with an increased risk. Selection of

Table 1. Mammographic Patters in 7,123 Women with 864 Breast Cancers
(Br Ca), with 206 Cancers Occurring 6 to 159 Months Following
a Normal Mammogram

Pattern	No. Women	Prevalent Br Ca	% Prevalent Br Ca	Incident Br Ca	% Incident Br Ca
N1	1,598	200	12.5	23	1.4
P1	1,045	170	16.3	20	1.9
P2	2,402	152	6.3	79	3.3
DY	2,078	136	6.5	84	4.0

those women destined to retain a glandular pattern with aging
would greatly reduce radiologists' concern with dense breasts.
The number of women with N1 pattern past 50 years of age was
double that of under 50 years, while the number in DY was
reduced by a factor of 4. This relative eightfold shift indicates
that with aging all breasts tend to assume uniformly a more
fatty appearance.

A disease in four subsets of the population with a similar
prevalence in each age group should have a similar incidence if

Table 2. Distribution of Total Breast Cancers (Br Ca), Prevalent Cancers
(Detected on Initial Examination) and Incident Cancers
(Detected Six Months or Longer After Noncancer Examination)

Age in Years	Total Cancers				Prevalent Cancers Per 1000 Women		Incident Cancers Per 1000 Women	
	N1, P1		P2, DY					
	No. Br Ca	Rate*	Br Ca	Rate*	N1, P1	P2, DY	N1, P1	P2, DY
30-34	4	6.0	18	16.3	6.0	16.3	0.0	0.0
35-39	15	18.4	24	17.9	17.2	11.9	1.2	6.0
40-44	40	40.7	79	47.8	40.7	33.9	0.0	13.9
45-49	51	48.9	69	52.2	44.1	28.7	4.8	23.5
50-54	47	55.7	62	81.7	54.5	36.9	1.2	44.8
55-59	50	70.0	64	120.8	53.8	73.6	15.2	47.2
60-64	48	82.2	66	168.4	73.6	109.7	8.6	58.7
65-69	47	112.4	34	134.4	105.3	87.0	7.2	47.4
70+	111	219.4	35	132.6	183.8	127.5	33.6	44.1
TOTAL	413	156.3	451	100.7	140.0	64.3	16.3	36.4

*Per 1000 women.

Table 3. Histopathologic Stage of the Cancers and Percentage
in Each Stage in Each Pattern

Pattern	Stage		
	0	1	2
N1	2 (9%)	13 (56%)	8 (35%)
P1	3 (15%)	11 (55%)	6 (30%)
P2	16* (20%)	44 (56%)	19 (24%)
DY	22† (26%)	36 (43%)	26 (31%)

*Includes 6 lobular carcinomas in situ.
†Includes 12 lobular carcinomas in situ.

followed adequately. During the first 36 months of follow-up
the incidence was shown to be eight times greater in P2, DY
than in N1, P1 but after that period the incidence became
similar. These two observations strongly suggest that breast
cancer is more difficult to detect by mammography in dense
breasts and many incident cancers are simply overlooked
prevalent cancers in dense breasts.

Despite an equal percentage of cancers classified histologically as stage 2, there is an increase in mortality among those
with DY pattern, compared to those with N1 pattern. This rate
would be almost doubled in DY if the lobular carcinomas in situ
were removed. All of the breast cancers were staged by the same
pathology department except three, and two of these were
reviewed by that same department. Fisher et al [10] demonstrated overlooked axillary lymph node metastases in one
quarter of cases of breast cancer studied by the routine
technique used by most pathologists and confirmed the

Table 4. Breast Cancer Mortality and Breast Pattern
in 206 Incident Cancers

Pattern	No. of Br Ca	Deaths	
		No.	Rate
N1	23	4	17%
P1	20	9	45%
P2	79*	17	22%
DY	84†	24	29%

*Includes 6 lobular carcinomas in situ.
†Includes 12 lobular carcinomas in situ.

fallibility of this approach. The assumption must be that there is a significant difference in actual stage of the cancers at diagnosis that is escaping histologic recognition.

No differences in the size of the tumor affecting staging (large tumors with no metastatic axillary nodes), its histologic type (more scirrhous cancers) or location (upper inner quadrant with greater chance of unknown internal mammary node metastases) could be demonstrated to explain the differences in mortality in DY and N1. Cancers are merely more advanced in dense breasts at the time of radiographic recognition, and our histologic staging is insensitive to some of the changes of this advanced disease.

Conclusions

Breast cancers are more frequent in older women with less glandular breasts. Cancers in glandular breasts are more difficult to detect by mammography and are more likely to remain prevalent than cancers in fatty breasts.

Incident breast cancers in dense breasts have a much poorer prognosis than those detected in more fatty breasts with comparable histologic staging, suggesting more advanced disease in dense breasts at detection.

References

1. Kelsey, J.L.: A review of the epidemiology of human breast cancer. Epidemiol. Rev. 1:74-109, 1979.
2. Egan, R.L.: Experience with mammography in a tumor institution. Radiology 75:894, 1960.
3. Qualheim, R.E. and Gall, E.A.: Breast carcinoma with multiple sites of origin. Cancer 10:460, 1957.
4. Warren, S.: The relation of "chronic mastitis" to carcinoma of the breast. Surg. Gynecol. Obstet. 71:257, 1940.
5. Egan, R.L., Ellis, J.T. and Powell, R.W.: Team approach to the study of diseases of the breast. Cancer 23:847, 1969.
6. Gallagher, H.S.: Correlation of radiological and pathological classifications in breast disease. Cancer Bull. 14:118, 1962.
7. Wolfe, J.N.: Risk for breast cancer development determined by mammographic parenchymal pattern. Cancer 37:2486, 1976.
8. Egan, R.L. and Mosteller, R.C.: Breast cancer mammography patterns. Cancer 40:2087, 1977.
9. Egan, R.L.: Estimated risk and occurrence of breast cancer in asymptomatic and minimally symptomatic patients. Cancer 43:871, 1979.

10. Fisher, E.R., Swamidoss, S., Lee, C.H. et al: Detection and significance of occult axillary node metastases in patients with invasive breast cancer. Cancer 42:2025, 1978.

Self-Evaluation Quiz

1. Wolfe reported a prospective study on radiographic parenchymal patterns.
   a) True
   b) False
2. Radiographically dense breasts occur much more frequently in younger women.
   a) True
   b) False
3. A prospective Emory University study has demonstrated that ductal hyperplasia is the only significant radiographic parenchymal pattern.
   a) True
   b) False
4. What percentage of total breast cancers are detected by mammography before 50 years of age?
   a) 1/4
   b) 1/3
   c) 1/2
   d) 2/3
5. Prevalent breast cancers were detected more frequently in:
   a) Fatty breasts
   b) Nodular breasts
   c) Dense breasts
6. Incident breast cancers were detected more frequently in:
   a) Fatty breasts
   b) Nodular breasts
   c) Dense breasts
7. Demonstration of increased incidence in dense breasts is due to:
   a) Difficulty of studying these breasts by mammography
   b) The fact that prevalent cancers are overlooked and become incident
   c) Both
8. In same-stage breast cancers, prognosis is poorer in:
   a) Fatty breasts
   b) Nodular breasts
   c) Denser breasts

9. In the Emory University study, the dense and fatty breasts
   in each age group had the same prevalence and incidence
   rates.
   a) True
   b) False
10. Your advice to the woman with clinically normal breasts
    that are radiographically dense should be to:
    a) Have an immediate excisional biopsy of the UOQ of
       each breast
    b) Proceed with prophylactic mastectomies without biopsy
    c) Both of the above
    d) None of the above

Answers on page 335.

Diaphanography: Transillumination of the Breast Revisited

Harold J. Isard, M.D.

Objective

The purpose of this paper is to assess the role of diaphanography as a noninvasive procedure for breast examination.

Transillumination of the breast was described more than 50 years ago, but its inadequacies and limitations in differentiating benign from malignant lesions of the breasts discouraged potential adherents and it failed to gain acceptance by the medical profession as a useful diagnostic test [1, 2]. The novel design of an apparatus by a Swedish company* utilizing a photographic technique to document and record the visual findings, comparable to spot filming during fluoroscopy, encouraged us to evaluate the technique, referred to as diaphanography, and to estimate its role as a noninvasive procedure in the examination of the breast.

The unit consists of a hand-held light source coupled to a 35-mm camera by an electronic unit that can vary the intensity of illumination. The light transmitter is so designed that no undue heat is generated. The photographic component of the examination makes use of a sensor, incorporated into the system, that is applied to the transilluminated breast to indicate

Harold J. Isard, M.D., F.A.C.R., Clinical Professor of Radiology, Temple University School of Medicine; and J. Gershon-Cohen Breast Clinic, Division of Radiology, Albert Einstein Medical Center, Philadelphia, Pa.

This study was supported in part by the Kapnek Charitable Trust.

*Sinus Medical Equipment.

the correct diaphragm setting of the camera for a 1/60 of a
second flash exposure. The camera itself is attached to a
wall-mounted arm that can be manipulated with ease. Infrared
film is recommended because it has the property of reproducing
with remarkable fidelity the reddish yellow color of the normal
breast tissues.

The examination is conducted in a darkened room and a
short period of dark adaptation of the eyes is necessary. With
the patient sitting on an examining table facing the examiner,
the light source is placed under the breast and moved about
until the entire breast is inspected. The other breast is similarly
examined. Without changing the patient's position, each breast
is photographed with the light source below and the camera
above. The patient is then placed on her side in the horizontal
position and the uppermost breast is transilluminated for
inspection, followed by photography with the light transmitter
applied to its under, or medial, surface. The examination is
expedited if both procedures are performed on one side before
having the patient turn for examination of the other breast. The
craniocaudal and lateral pictures have been adopted as routine
and they are comparable to the standard mammographic
images. Whereas it has been stated in the literature that the light
source should be as close as possible to a suspected breast
lesion, it is obvious that this is not correct. A mass within the
breast will be projected to best advantage, with less diffusion of
the shadow, when it is closer to the surface being photographed
and farther from the light source.

Initially, in order to gain experience and establish interpre-
tative criteria, investigation was generally restricted to symptomatic patients or those in whom mammographic findings
were abnormal. The usual yellow-reddish color will be dependent upon the size of the breast and the relative amounts of fat
and fibroglandular tissues, while skin pigment apparently is of
little significance. Abnormalities can be recognized by shadows,
color differences and vascular aberrations. Well-circumscribed
opacities commonly found by mammography are rarely as well
defined by diaphanography unless they are on the skin surface
or immediately beneath it. Cysts containing clear fluid are
usually quite lucent, benign fibroadenomas may be reddish to
brown, cancers are frequently darker brown with indistinct or

irregular margins, while hemorrhage in the breast is practically black. Benign fibrocystic disease is usually suggested by a deeper red color. Vascular abnormalities consisting of alterations in caliber, configuration and numbers of vessels may be the predominant findings in certain malignancies. It is important to note that small calcifications have not been identified.

Some of these criteria can be recognized during diaphanoscopy — the visual inspection — but final interpretation should await review of the documented images in order to compare the two breasts, particularly when the lesions are less obvious and the changes are subtle.

Results

Approximately 300 patients have been examined, and of the first 100 subjected to biopsy or aspiration, the diaphanographic findings of the 53 histologically proven malignancies were analyzed (Table 1). Concurrently with diaphanography, physical examination was performed and mammographic and thermographic studies were made. In all instances the decision for intervention was based upon the clinical and mammographic findings. Five cases were considered unsatisfactory for interpretation by diaphanography because of poor technique, or either a breast too small for adequate examination or excessive tissue density. Five cases were considered normal by diaphanography and three were indeterminate. Forty patients, or 75% of the group, had abnormal findings in accord with the criteria previously described. The level of accuracy in this group of symptomatic patients is somewhat less than that of other investigators in Sweden and Italy, who reported accuracy levels of 90% to 96% [3-5].

Table 1. Diaphanography:
53 Cancers Histologically Confirmed

Diaphanographic Interpretation	Number	%
Normal	5	9.4
Abnormal	40	75.4
Indeterminate	3	5.3
Technically unsatisfactory	5	9.4

Conclusions

While diaphanography is an attractive modality, it has some limitations. With present techniques it does not appear to be suitable for screening asymptomatic women, primarily because of its lack of identification of calcification. Very small breasts and extremely dense breasts are difficult to examine. Future innovations in camera automation can obviate errors in setting exposure factors and thereby reduce the number of unsatisfactory examinations. Infrared film requires special processing which may not be readily available. The obvious advantage of diaphanography is the fact that it is a safe, noninvasive procedure that can be used in the examining physician's office in conjunction with physical examination. The recorded images can be filed for comparison with subsequent examinations. In the evaluation of obvious clinical lesions and the differentiation of large cysts from tumors, the experienced observer may limit the examination to diaphanoscopy. For the radiologist diaphanography is another dimension that supplements mammography.

Correlation with physical findings and/or mammography was achieved in 75% of 53 cases of breast cancer. As in other imaging disciplines, technical proficiency and skillful interpretation are required to attain a satisfactory level of diagnostic accuracy.

References

1. Cutler, M.: Transillumination as an aid in the diagnosis of breast lesions. Surg. Gynecol. Obstet. 48:721, 1929.
2. Cheatle, G.L. and Cutler, M.: Tumours of the Breast. Philadelphia:J. B. Lippincott Co., 1930, p. 323.
3. Di Maggio, C. and Pescarini, L.: Use of transillumination in the diagnosis of breast disorders. Institute of Radiology of Padua University, Italy, 1975.
4. Ohlsson, B., Gundersen, J. and Nilsson, D.M.: Diaphanography — A method of evaluation of the tissues in the female breast. Veberods Medical Center and Central Hospital, Sweden, 1977.
5. Wallberg, H. and Alveryd, A.: Investigation with diaphanography, mammography and cytological examination in the diagnosis of breast cancer. Report of Huddinge Hospital, Sweden, 1978.

Self-Evaluation Quiz

1. Diaphanography utilizes a photographic technique to document and record visual findings of transillumination.

   a) True
   b) False

2. _____ film best reproduces the color of normal breast tissue.
   a) Low-dose
   b) Xerographic
   c) Infrared
   d) Ultrafast screen

3. The light source should be as close as possible to the suspected lesion.
   a) True
   b) False

4. Diaphanography is not suitable for screening asymptomatic women.
   a) True
   b) False

Answers on page 335.

Flexi-Therm™:
Vacuum-Contoured, Liquid Crystal, Dynamic Breast Thermoangiography as an Aid to Mammography in the Detection of Breast Cancer

Rubem Pochaczevsky, M.D. and Phillip H. Meyers, M.D.

Objective

New thermographic equipment is introduced in the form of liquid crystals embedded in flexible, transparent, elastomeric sheaths which may be vacuum contoured to any breast. Dynamic thermoangiography, a new physiological method of performing thermography with these liquid crystal sheaths, is presented. Thermographic changes are recorded during active skin cooling and rewarming with liquid crystals in situ. The new system eliminates skin preparation previously required. Preliminary results appear to show good correlation with conventional telethermography. Vascular as well as thermal pathology is accentuated with rich, high-contrast, thermographically calibrated color patterns. The new system is relatively inexpensive, simple to operate, and may be suited to a program for the detection of breast cancer.

Introduction

Liquid crystals are special compounds which are usually cholesterol derivatives. They show strong optical molecular

Rubem Pochaczevsky, M.D., F.A.C.R., Department of Radiology, Long Island Jewish Hillside Medical Center, New Hyde Park, N.Y.; and Phillip H. Meyers, M.D., Clinical Associate Professor of Radiology, Tulane Medical School, New Orleans, La.

Reprinted from *Clinical Radiology* 30:405-411, 1979.

rotatory power and selectively reflect polarized light in a narrow region of wavelengths. Their molecular arrangement, however, is altered with temperature change. It is this latter property which results in a specific color temperature response which is utilized in color thermography [1, 2].

The adaptation of liquid crystals to thermography had, until recently, been hampered by the necessity of preparing the skin with a black, water-based paint prior to its being sprayed with the liquid crystals [1, 3]. Although plastic plates were subsequently developed which obviated skin preparation or spraying [4, 5], difficulties in achieving adequate thermographic examination of the entire breast persisted, since the plates which contained the liquid crystals were unwieldy and rigid.

This paper is a work-in-progress report of an ongoing study describing the feasibility of a new thermographic technique. It does not purport to be a statistical analysis of its merits. The new thermographic technique employs flexible, transparent, elastomeric plastic sheaths which house the liquid crystals. Since the thermally sensitive liquid crystals are now contained within a flexible housing, they can be contoured to any breast shape. A newly incorporated vacuum system further assures uniform skin contact.

Material

The case material consists of 174 consecutive examinations in two institutions performed in approximately one year. All patients were symptomatic or at high risk for breast cancer. Mammography was performed on all patients.

Apparatus

The apparatus consists of liquid crystal sets contained in elastomeric sheaths,* a vacuum system and a photographic camera.

Liquid crystals are supplied in five or more temperature ranges. They are incorporated within newly developed elastomeric transparent Flexi-Therm* sheaths measuring 30 cm wide

---

*Flexi-Therm^{TM} Elastomeric liquid crystal sheaths and apparatus supplied by Flexi-Therm, Inc., 117 Magnalia Avenue, Westbury, NY 11590, U.S.A. (516-334-1980).

by 90 cm long (12 × 36 in). A vacuum system assures their intimate contact with any size breast. They are additionally fitted with Velcro closure straps.

A Polaroid camera (Model CU-5) utilizing 108-type film, equipped with an electronic flash system and cross-field polarized filters to reduce glare, serves to record the color thermograms. Alternatively, a 35-mm camera with a similar flash system may be used.

Liquid crystals have demonstrated an accurate and reliable color response to specific temperature ranges. The lowest temperature is displayed as a dark brown color. This changes with progressive temperature elevation, from brown to red, green and blue. The highest temperature is indicated by a dark blue color. Liquid crystal sheaths are progressively numbered 31°, 32°, 33° and 35°, corresponding to their median Celsius temperature range (Table 1).

Conduct of the Examination

The skin temperature is stabilized by uncovering the breasts and axillae in a cool room (approximately 20°C) for approximately ten minutes. Selection of the proper liquid crystal sheath with the widest color display is made by wrapping a midrange 33°C sheath about the patient as noted below. If brown colors predominate, the skin temperature is too cold for that particular sheath. A 32° or 31°C sheath is then used. If blue colors predominate, the skin temperature is too warm and a 34° or 35°C sheath is used. The appropriate liquid crystal sheath is then wrapped around the patient and secured posteriorly by means of Velcro straps. Velcro shoulder straps provide additional sheath immobilization. The vacuum valve is

Table 1. Typical Liquid Crystal Elastomeric Temperature Calibrations (°C)

No.	Dark Brown	Light Brown	Dark Red	Light Red	Green	Light Blue	Dark Blue
32	31.3	31.6	31.9	32.2	32.4	33.2	35.0
33	32.0	32.3	32.7	33.6	33.7	34.6	36.0
34	32.9	33.2	33.4	34.0	34.2	35.3	36.4

These color temperature calibrations permit simultaneous determinations of temperature differentials ($\Delta T°$) in comparable regions of both breasts.

then connected to a suction pump which establishes a vacuum within seconds. Filming is then started and standard frontal (Fig. 1) and both oblique views are taken. The entire study may be performed in an average time of 15 minutes.

Dynamic Thermography

An extension of this technique is the possibility of dynamically observing the effects of cooling on the thermogram [1, 4]. Observation and documentation during cooling and spontaneous rewarming constitute a physiological approach which may yield useful information. We have included this dynamic phase of the study in most of our examinations without significant prolongation (an average of five minutes). Cooling is done by means of a fan and may be performed with the liquid crystal sheath in situ. Disappearance and reappearance of colors is thereby dynamically documented. Alternatively, more intense cooling may be obtained by spraying the skin of the breasts, axillae and inframammary regions with alcohol which is then evaporated with a fan for one minute prior to liquid crystal sheath application. Filming is then done during the course of progressive skin cooling with the fan operating and the sheath in situ. The fan is then eliminated, and the rewarming phase is photographed. Any geographic zone of thermal dissimilarity or vascular discrepancy between the two breasts is thereby dynamically documented.

Dynamic thermography proved to be valuable in documenting the thermal symmetry of normal breasts. Spurious increases in temperature appeared to disappear with cooling, while abnormal elevations remained localized, persisted longer and showed an ability to reappear more promptly after cooling (Fig. 2). Abnormal vascular patterns may also become more prominent after cooling.

Correlation with Mammography and Conventional Telethermography

Twelve histologically proven breast carcinomas were found in 11 of 174 patients examined with liquid crystal thermography. One case had bilateral carcinomas. All were demonstrated by mammography (Figs. 2 and 3). All cases also had

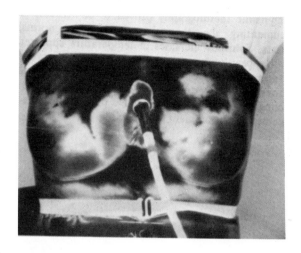

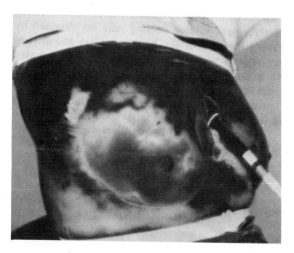

FIG. 1. Normal patient. Frontal and right oblique views. Note symmetric multicolor thermal and vascular patterns. (Original paper was printed in full color. For copies of the original reprints, please write Phillip H. Meyers, M.D., 401 Emerald St., New Orleans, LA 70124. Telephone [504] 895-7755.)

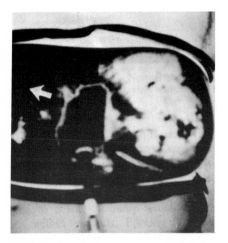 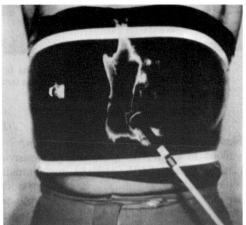

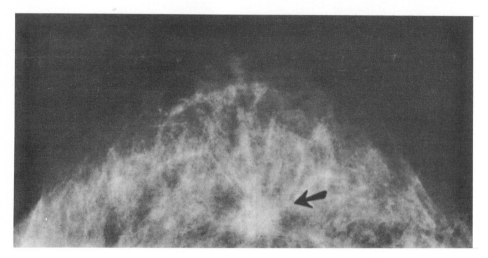

FIG. 2. Case 2, carcinoma of left breast. Forty-year-old female with a 2 ×
3-cm, ill-defined, superior lateral quadrant mass noted on routine clinical
examination. *Top left*, Precooling discloses bilateral hyperthermic breasts
(blue colors) more marked on the left. *Top right*, Postcooling demonstrated lowered right breast temperature but persistently high left breast
temperature. Note abnormally dilated vessels (*arrow*) displayed as thick
blue streaks in the inner upper quadrant. *Bottom*, Mammogram shows a
1.0 × 0.5-cm tumor in this region. At surgery an infiltrating ductal
carcinoma was found, with one of 24 axillary nodes reported as positive.

abnormal liquid crystal thermograms (Fig. 2) and abnormal conventional telethermograms (Fig. 3) in every instance when the latter were performed (five patients). Conventional tele-thermography ("Thermiscope") was performed, together with liquid crystal thermography, on 124 patients. Our initial preliminary impression, based on these 124 cases, suggests a good correlation between liquid crystal thermography and conventional telethermography (Fig. 3). Statistical analysis of these two thermographic methods awaits the accumulation of additional case material and longer follow-up. However, Gautherie et al [6, 7] had previously reported a good correlation between liquid crystal thermography and conventional telethermography in various clinical settings.

Contrary to conventional telethermography, liquid crystal colors vary in a nonlinear, parabolic fashion. Therefore, by selecting the crystal with the proper temperature range, color contrast is enhanced and findings may be even more dramatic-ally displayed than in conventional telethermography. Liquid crystal studies emphasize vascular patterns by means of bold, contrasting, thermographically calibrated blue or green colors. The resultant thermoangiogram is particularly advantageous for superficial vessel analysis (Fig. 3).

Liquid crystals may also be better suited to the examination of pendulous breasts, which are notoriously difficult to study with conventional telethermography [8], even in the supine position. The vacuum-contoured sheaths effectively lift the breasts, permitting their inferior aspects to be cooled and studied. The vacuum technique proved equally efficacious in the examination of large breasts.

Since a major portion of the examination is conducted with the liquid crystal sheath in situ, there is less infringement on patient modesty than with telethermography.

Thermoangiography

Feldman [9, 10] performed angiography of the breasts and demonstrated abnormal angiographic findings in breast cancers. Due to enhanced vascular definition with color contrast, a variety of abnormal thermographic vascular patterns have been noted in association with mammary malignancy. Tricoire et al [11-13] reported a radial distribution of vessels emanating

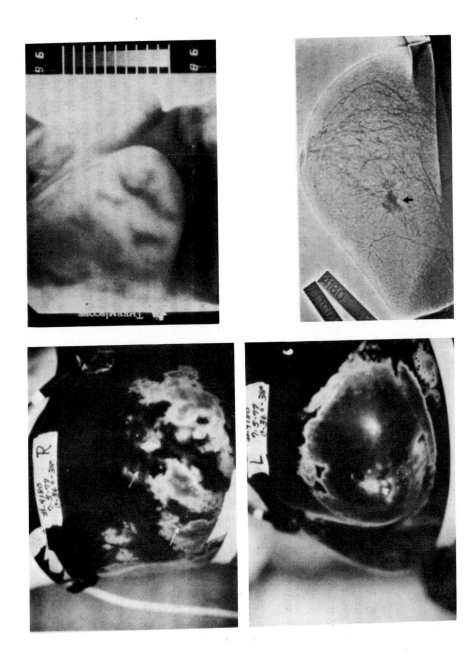

FIG. 3. Case 4, carcinoma of right breast. Fifty-eight-year-old female noted thickened skin along medial aspect of right breast for three weeks. *Top left*, Liquid crystal thermography of right breast. A radial "spoke wheel" pattern with a central hollow loop is formed by abnormally prominent vessels, displayed as blue curvilinear lines (*arrows*) surrounding a brown, relatively cool, central area. The predominance of blue and green colors throughout the right breast indicates an increased temperature. *Top right*, Conventional telethermogram shows similar findings with vessels displayed as black curvilinear lines. *Bottom left*, Left breast shows no abnormal vessels. The predominance of dark brown colors indicates that the left breast is significantly cooler than the right. *Bottom right*, Right breast xeroradiograph shows a spiculated mass (*arrow*) in the superior medial quadrant. At surgery, an infiltrating ductal carcinoma was found with no axillary metastases. Comment: This case illustrates that a strongly positive thermogram confirmed the presence of a breast lesion and indicates that thermographic findings are not necessarily confined to or superimposed on the quadrant occupied by the lesion.

from a central loop or core. The latter may be relatively
hypothermic and, therefore, appear hollow, or relatively hyperthermic with a central, solid-appearing area of increased
temperature. A "spoke wheel" silhouette is simulated in both
instances, one with a central hollow loop and the other with a
seemingly solid center. Simpler radial arrangements composed
of fewer vessels may assume the shapes of three or four pointed
"vascular stars" with rays emanating from a central but smaller
locus than those of the spoke wheels. Other varied converging
configurations, parallel or "railroad track" patterns as well as
solitary, "club-shaped" abnormal accentuations of single vessels,
were also described. We were able to identify the above-
mentioned abnormal vascular patterns in most of our breast
carcinomas (Figs. 1-3).

Discussion

The proposed new technique of liquid crystal thermography
could serve as a useful adjunct in a program for the detection of
breast cancer for the following reasons:

1. Apparent good correlation with conventional telethermography.
2. Low Cost. The entire apparatus costs less than $6000 or
   a small fraction of the cost of a conventional thermographic unit. This permits its routine use, either as a
   prepalpation study or in conjunction with mammography in small hospitals and physicians' offices.
3. Simple apparatus. Total equipment consists solely of
   crystal sheaths, a camera and accessories, and a vacuum
   pump.
4. Easy to operate.
5. Easy to store. The entire unit can be stored in a 1.0 ×
   0.5 × 0.5-m cupboard space.
6. Mobile. It can be easily transported and utilized in
   various locations.
7. Noninvasive. No exposure to radiation.
8. Color contrast. Liquid crystals dramatically accentuate
   pathological findings with a rich, high-contrast, thermographically calibrated color display. Vascular abnormalities are particularly well delineated.

Conclusion

Dynamic thermoangiography with liquid crystals has yielded additional useful information in our current case material (Fig. 2) and appears worthy of the additional minutes required for cooling, especially in equivocal cases.

Abnormal vascular patterns described in the European literature [11-13], obtained with liquid crystal thermography, were reproduced in most of our cases (Figs. 2 and 3). Although it has yet to become firmly established, liquid crystal thermography may prove to be a useful adjunct, together with clinical examination and mammography, in screening for breast cancers.

Acknowledgments

The technical contributions of Mr. Seymour Katz and Ms. Theodora Masterfano are gratefully acknowledged.

References

1. Archer, F.: Utilisation des cristaux liquides en thermographie medicale. These Medecine, Strasbourg, 1969, no. 53.
2. Crissey, J.J., Gordy, E., Fergason, J.L. and Lyman, R.B.: A new technique for the demonstration of skin temperature patterns. J. Invest. Dermatol. 43:89-91, 1964.
3. Logan, W.W. and Lind, B.: Improved liquid cholesterol ester crystal thermography of the breast. J. Surg. Oncol. 8:363-368, 1976.
4. Barth, V., Muller, R., Beininger, H.K. and Wollgens, P.: Klinik, mammographi, zytologie, stanzbiopsie und plattenthermographie in der erweiterten mammadiagnostik. Dtsch. Med. Wochenschr. 99:175-180, 1974.
5. Fochem, K. and Pflanzer, K.: Plate thermography: A new method of mammary examination [preliminary report]. Wein. Klin. Wochenschr. 86 [21]:664-666, 1974.
6. Gautherie, M., Quenneville, Y. and Gros, C.: Cholesteric thermography. Sheets of liquid crystal. Clinical, pharmacological and physiological applications. Comparisons with infrared thermography. Patholog. Biol. 22 [7]:553-566, 1974.
7. Gautherie, M., Quenneville, Y., Rempp, C. and Gros, C.: Valeur informative comparée de la téléthermographie [infrarogue] et de la thermographie de contact [cristaux liquides] in senologie. J. Radiol. Electrol. Med. Nucl. 56 [suppl. 1]:316-318, 1975.

8. Stark, A.M. and Way, S.: The use of thermovision in the detection of early breast cancer. Cancer 33:1664-1670, 1974.
9. Feldman, F.: Angiography of cancer of the breast. Cancer 23:803-808, 1969.
10. Feldman, F., Habif, D.V., Fleming, R.J. et al: Arteriography of the breast. Radiology 80:1053-1061, 1967.
11. Tricoire, J., Mariel, L. and Amiel, J.P.: Thermography and the diagnosis of small breast tumours. Nouv. Presse Med. 2 [17]:1117-1119, 1973.
12. Tricoire, J., Mariel, L. and Amiel, J.P.: La thermographie en plaque dans l'étude des cancers du sein. Apport pronostique et thérapeutique. Nouv. Presse Med. 4 [1]:50-52, 1975.
13. Tricoire, J., Mariel, L. Amiel, J.P. et al: Thermographie en plaque de 300 malades atteintes d'affections variees du sein. Presse Med. 78:2183-2186, 1970.

Self-Evaluation Quiz

Vacuum-contoured, liquid crystal Flexi-Therm contact breast thermography will help you:

1. To identify those high-risk patients who require mammograms for correlation or clarification.
    a) True
    b) False
2. To examine younger patients.
    a) True
    b) False
3. When you need a deciding factor to initiate a biopsy where palpatory and/or mammographic findings were equivocal.
    a) True
    b) False
4. To identify low-risk patients for periodic clinical observation and establish follow-up procedures.
    a) True
    b) False
5. As a prepalpation test to attract attention to areas of increased heat emission which may harbor malignant foci.
    a) True
    b) False
6. To identify high-risk patients who would require follow-up breast profiles.
    a) True
    b) False

7. To identify patients with inflammatory carcinomas which may require special treatment.
   a) True
   b) False
8. To follow patients with treated breast carcinoma to detect new tumor developments.
   a) True
   b) False

Answers on page 335.

The Physiology of the Breast by Cholesteric Plate Analysis

William B. Hobbins, M.D.

Objectives

1. To increase understanding of anatomical, physiological and pathological conditions of the breast in relation to blood flow as measured by infrared thermal monitoring.
2. To demonstrate the effect on classifying "aggressive disease" from "limited potential disease" in breast cancer on the basis of doubling time, measured by thermal content of colorgrams. This should be used in designing treatment programs in these subsets and can be determined preoperatively.

Introduction

The purpose of this paper is to present the observations of the physiology of the breast as recorded by thermal surface study.

The biophysiology of the breast can be expressed as blood flow [1-3]. The best measurement of blood flow of the breast is thermography, according to Love [4]. Draper stated in 1971, after a thermobiology engineering study: "The observed thermal patterns over malignant tumors of small size (less than .8 cm) are evidently due chiefly to some effect of the tumor on the blood flow in the superficial veins" [3, 5]. In 1953, Schwamm observed the viscerocutaneous reflexes as evidenced by infrared monitoring [6], and Lawson first reported the thermal infrared reaction of breast pathology in 1956 [7].

William B. Hobbins, M.D., President, Wisconsin Breast Cancer Detection Foundation, Madison, Wis.

Monitoring of the infrared emmission of the breast surface and thereby, indirectly, the blood flow of the breast is actually a reflection of the many influences on the sympathetic nervous system. This is the control of the peripheral vascular blood flow. We must, as we evaluate thermal responses, recognize the major control — the nervous system. This is to say, pain, anoxia, products of metabolism, toxic and physiologic substances all manifest their thermal effect in the breast through the sympathetic response, as do most pathologic conditions [8].

Method

The findings recorded here are a result of analysis of 78,000 thermograms processed by Wisconsin Breast Cancer Detection Foundation, Inc. from 1972 to 1978. This background material has been further defined by accurate examination with choles-teric plate technology since 1977 [9]. Some 21,000 colorgrams, which are the resultant recording of a reflected image from a cholesteric plate placed against the breast, were analyzed with regard to physiopathologic condition of the patient examined and have been classified as to thermal response. The literature was used as a yardstick to confirm the observations and, as such, is recorded as well.

Results

Anatomic

Anatomically, there are three major factors: size, vascular anomaly and skin abnormalities.

Since the thermal response is a comparative study as to symmetry with a contralateral side, size becomes a large factor. As a general rule in a given patient, the smaller breast is warmer, whereas the larger breast is the colder. Quantity of parenchyma of the breasts is usually equal, and size disparity is most often a difference in fatty tissue which insulates the thermal conduction even from the convection portion of the dispersing process [10].

Superficial varicosities of the skin will increase apparent vascularity and, when asymmetrical, can lead to a false interpretation of the significance of the initial colorgam [8, 11].

The surface of the skin of the breast may also influence the thermal imagery of the breast. Congenital lesions such as hemangioma are generally warmer than the surrounding area. Infections of the skin, such as boils, carbuncles, pimples and some rashes, show increased infrared activity. The center of the larger inflammatory lesions may be cool as a result of decreased blood flow due to necrosis, devascularization and edema.

New growths of the skin usually have increased thermal response. Gautherie has stated that melanoma can be divided on this basis into classes of biological significance of the malignancy: the hotter the colorgram, the more serious the prognosis [8].

Physiologic

The physiologic observations of the cholesteric analysis profile (CAP) test are divided into four major groups: primary nervous system, hormonal system, environmental manipulation (chemical and physical) and pathologic processes.

Nervous System. The somatic nervous system can influence the breast thermal response. Cases of spinal scoliosis have caused unilateral hyperthermia or hypothermia. Fractured ribs with intercostal nerve damage have been known to cause galactorrhea and to be associated with hyperthermia [12]. The visceral aspect of the breast, the acinar and ductal tissue, will cause local thermic changes due to reflex sympathetic stimulus. Distention, or incomplete involution, with cyst formation, will often cause a cold thermal response through vasoconstriction of the area [13]. This is associated with the most common cause of mastodynia, visceral reflexive pain secondary to cystic mastopathy.

The paresthesia of sympathetic stimulation is usually associated with a hot spot on a colorgram. Many theories exist to explain this burning, stinging pain. Again, a sympathetic reflexive pain is thought to occur in anoxic processes or where there is incomplete metabolism or some type of immune reaction. Kiricuta of Romania has increased hyperthermia in breast cancer by administration of IV glucose [14]. This may be evidence of the above metabolic process since the burning, stinging pain has a high correlation with breast cancer and hyperthermia.

Stress to the nervous system may cause a vasoconstriction. Placing the hands in ice water for 45 seconds will cause the normal breast thermal response to decrease by 1° C. Immersion of one or both hands will cause an equal or bilateral symmetrical response in the normal person. In the presence of an active tumor, in response to such stress, the hyperthermia is increased. This paradoxical action is explained by the fact that the heat source, the cancer and its neovascularity, does not have the nervous control of normal vessels. This is further understood when one studies the rationale of angiotensin injections intra-arterially to enhance the demonstration of renal tumor. This causes constriction of the non-neoplastic arteries and allows more selective filling of the tumor with contrast media [15].

This may not separate abscesses from cancer in view of the fact that the neovascularity of granulation tissue is also unresponsive to vasoconstrictive drugs [16].

Hormonal System. The hormonal group of physiologic responses is among the more interesting. They always affect the breasts symmetrically if the breast tissue is healthy. This is important to understand when considering pathology. Early in puberty, the parenchymal growth shows an equal nonvascular pattern. As the breasts mature, vascularity increases and then decreases once again at menopause. During adult life, pregnancy and lactation create a vascular hypertrophy (dilatation) with increased hyperthermia. It should be noted that nursing can create a unilateral cooling and asymmetry due to loss of heat content of the suckled milk. It is best to image and observe nursing women in a prenursing period (four-hour abstinence) or with both breasts suckled for an equal time. Areas of hyperthermia in a nursing breast or clinical suspicion which does not change upon nursing should be regarded with increased concern.

Manipulation of the body with BCP or hormone replacement can be monitored by the CAP test. If the replacement is estrogen-dominant, the result will be a rise in hPRL serum prolactin. This will result in progesterone reduction [12]. The hypervascular thermal change will then occur. This is similar to pregnancy and lactation, but is not as extensive. Only 20% of BCP patients will show this change when CAP tested before institution and then compared 90 days later. Also, when the progesterone-deficient state is treated by progesterone applied to breast, the thermal signal is returned to the expected normal pattern.

Other conditions, such as Chiari-Frommel, Ahunada-del Castillo and Forbes-Albright syndromes, have a similar thermal response. Only two cases of spontaneous amenorrhea and galactorrhea without pituitary adenoma have been seen by the author. One of these cases may be an adenoma in regression. Galactorrhea and hypothyroidism have been seen, and when treated with thyroid, the hypervascularity of the upper halves of the breasts regresses on colorgram.

Environmental Factors. Environmental changes in the physiology of the breast have been observed. The common thermal response is that of progesterone deficiency (relative) and may or may not be associated with galactorrhea [13]. Any drug that will increase prolactin and thus decrease progesterone production will result in the characteristic colorgram [12]. Examples of these drugs are the phenothiazides, tricyclic antidepressants, meprobamate, haloperidol, alpha-methyldopa, reserpine, amphetamines and isoniazid, as well as sympathetic blocking agents such as Inderal and others. On the colorgrams, the changes from these drugs are seen in the increased vascularity and hyperthermia in the upper halves of the breasts. This effect is always symmetrical. When there is an observed change in the colorgram since a previous recording, without explanation, the patient's new medications should be considered for possible explanation, if the response is symmetrical.

Pathologic Factors. Up to this point, the majority of the conditions described cause a bilateral symmetrical response in the breasts and are observed in the colorgram in this fashion. The fourth group of conditions that affect the physiology of the breast is the pathologic ones. These usually affect only one breast or an isolated area of that breast. It must be remembered that the observed response is not always in direct position with the pathology due to vascular drainage of the segmental anatomy of the breast.

There are many pathologic conditions of the breast which change the physiology as monitored by colorgrams [17]. The major classes are (1) inflammation, (2) trauma, (3) mastopathy, and (4) neoplasia. The blood flow of the breast is changed by every pathologic condition and can be studied with a CAP test.

1. *Inflammation*. Breast infection, whether deep or superficial, usually brings forth increased blood flow. This will be observed as hyperthermia in the area and may be limited to one quadrant or affect the entire breast, depending on the severity. Tuberculosis of the breast has been seen to cause an abnormal CAP test result [18].

2. *Trauma*. Trauma to the breast will respond in different ways. When the injury includes the chest wall and associated nerves, there may be a hyperthermic response initially. Vasoconstriction may occur as the result of sympathetic reflex and may be observed as segmental cold response on the CAP test in other cases. Fat necrosis and hematomas are generally observed as cold segmental findings. This is as would be expected, due to decreased blood flow in the area and often surrounding edema.

3. *Mastopathy*. The pathophysiologic breast changes in benign conditions of breast function and repair are generally cold, as discussed elsewhere. Fibrocystic conditions, sclerosing adenosis and other such normally occurring changes will have segmental vasoconstriction associated with reflex pain when active. The heat of metabolic activity is usually suppressed by cystic spaces and dense fibrosis and the resulting reduced blood flow. It should be stated that the resultant cold unilateral response has frequently led to an interpretation of hyperthermia in the other breasst, which was normal or not showing a similar activity at the time. Colorgrams must always be interpreted in light of known clinical findings in order to increase the significance of the study [[11, 19-22].

4. *Neoplasia*. Neoplasia, as observed by CAP, is probably the most important. It must be stated that thermal response is directly proportional to the biologic significance of the tumor [17, 19-21, 23-25]. The increase in blood flow as evidenced by hyperthermia and hypervascularity correlates with degree of biologic activity [1, 11, 17, 20, 26]. Whether this is directly from the metabolism or indirectly from host immune response, it correlates without respect to size of tumor mass — 65% of <1-cm malignant tumors have shown various degrees of hyperthermia [17, 21, 22, 27, 28]. On the other hand, inflammatory carcinoma has thermal disturbance observed by CAP of greater than 6° C when contralaterally compared with the normal breast.

Tumor growth has been studied extensively, and doubling time of the cell mass has been used as a measure of biologic significance [29]. Mammography has aided the in vivo observations of growth. Doubling times of 40 days up to 500 days have been measured [8, 17, 26]. The blood flow is now known to be directly related to this doubling as observed by thermal response. Fournier and others find a direct parallel between thermal gradient and doubling time by mammography [26]. Although the bioengineers cannot explain this observation on the basis of metabolism of cell mass alone, the observation is consistent [1]. The influence of the autoimmune reaction of the body also must play a role and be reflected in blood flow as the organism attempts to control the cancerous process. Influence of stimulation by thalamic hormonal changes in defense will also reflect on the thermal biology of the host.

Benign neoplasias, such as fibroadenoma, will often show a mild hyperthermal response. The more rapidly appearing and faster enlarging ones are the hottest.

In malignant neoplasia, size of tumor is not the apparent physiologic reason for the observed hyperthermia, as previously mentioned [1, 2, 5]. A large 4-cm medullary or scirrhous cancer most often will be cold, and a 0.5-cm nonpalpable intraductal cancer can be observed to have a $3°$ ΔT hyperthermia, hypervascular CAP test. It has been confirmed by many, starting with Williams [30], then Gautherie and Gros [8], Amalric, Spitalier and Giraud [11] and others, that thermal biologic observation is an accurate method of determining prognosis for survival. This relationship of blood flow and thermal gradient is a dynamic measurement of the significance of biogenesis of the neoplasia to the host.

Henderson et al, in the *New England Journal of Medicine*, state: "There are at least two different populations of patients with breast cancer: one in which the tumor grows large within a breast without either regional or distant metastasis and another in which distant metastasis occurs before there is extensive growth within the breast" [31].

He further states that the group of patients with the best prognosis, "clinical stage A with no nodal involvement really consists of three subgroups: those with aggressive disease that has limited local growth but early metastasis ('aggressive disease'); those with moderately aggressive disease that has limited local growth and has not yet metastasized; and those with limited local growth that may have been present for some time without metastasis and has a limited future potential for metastasis ('limited potential disease')."

He further states that the group of patients with the best prognosis. "clinical stage A with no nodal involvement really consists of three subgroups: those with aggressive disease that has limited local growth but early metastasis ('aggressive disease'); those with moderately aggressive disease that has limited local growth that may have been present for some time without metastasis and have a limited future potential for metastasis ('limited potential disease')."

Fox has stated that if all of these patients are treated in the same manner, it is possible that those with "aggressive disease" will be undertreated and those with "limited potential disease" will be overtreated [32]. The specialized Breast Cancer Treatment Center in Marseille, France, has for ten years designed its therapeutic (preoperative) program on the basis of thermography. Amalric and Spitalier have over 1600 cases so treated with excellent results [11, 20].

The thermobiology of the breast, as observed by CAP test, gives the best pretreatment assessment of the suspect lesion and has been shown to correlate with nodal status and survival. All prospective studies of breast cancer should be qualified and measured by thermography so as to assess the thermobiology of the morphologic tumor.

Conclusion

It can be stated that thermography monitors blood flow of the breast and thereby records and assesses any condition which influences this physiologically. Anatomic and physiologic conditions can be differentiated with colorgrams. A significant use is that it differentiates biologically significant cancers from less significant ones and can help in the establishment of treatment protocols.

In the long-range view, much will be gained in understanding of the physiopathology of the breast by these noninvasive observations and recordings of thermal biology.

References

1. Chato, J.C.: Measurement of thermal properties of growing tumors. Proc. N.Y. Acad. Sci. 335:67-85, 1980.
2. Bowman, H.F.: The bio-heat transfer equation and discrimination of thermally significant vessels. Proc. N.Y. Acad Sci. 335:155-160, 1980.
3. Nelsson, S.K.: Surface temperatures over an implanted artificial heat source. Phys. Med. Biol. 19 (5):677-691, 1974.
4. Love, T.J.: Thermography as an indicator of blood perfusion. Proc. N.Y. Acad. Sci. 335:429-437, 1980.
5. Draper, J.: Skin temperature distribution over veins and tumors. Phys. Med. Biol. 16 (4):645-654, 1971.
6. Schwamm, E.: The infra-red radiation of the man. Hippocrates, Dec. 1953.
7. Lawson, R.: Implications of surface temperatures in the diagnosis of breast cancer. Can. Med. Assoc. J. 75:309-310, 1956.
8. Gautherie, M. and Gros, C.M.: Contribution of Infrared Thermography to Early Diagnosis, Pre-therapeutic Prognosis and Post-irradiation Follow-up of Breast Carcinomas. Strasbourg, France: Laboratory of Electroradiology, Faculty of Medicine, Louis Pasteur University, 1976.
9. Hobbins, W.B.: Comparison of telethermography and cholesteric plate thermography in breast thermal examinations. Presented at 3rd European Thermographic Society Congress, Barcelona, Spain, Sept. 24, 1978. Acta Thermograph. (In press.)
10. Volker, B.: Atlas of Disease of the Breast. Chicago:Year Book Medical Publishers, 1979.
11. Amalric, R., Spitalier, J.M., Giraud, D. et al: Thermography in diagnosis of breast disease. Bibl. Radiol. 6:65-76, 1975.
12. Archer, D.F.: Current concepts of prolactin physiology in normal and abnormal conditions. Fertil. Steril. 28 (2):125-131, 1977.
13. LaFaye, C. and Aubert, B.: The action of local progesterone therapy on benign mastopathies: A study of 500 cases. Breast 5 (1):9-13, 1979.
14. Kiricuta, I.: The value of the tumoral hyperthermia test provoked by administration of glucose in clinical exploration of the breast cancer. Acta Thermograph. 3 (3):118-120, 1978.
15. Reuter and Redman: Gastrointestinal Angiography. Philadelphia:W. B. Saunders, 1979, pp. 271-273.
16. Doppman, J.F., Fried, L.S. and Dibhero, G.: Absent constrictive response of wound vessels to intra-arterial vasopressors: Angiographic observations. Radiology 93:57, 1969.
17. Gautherie, M. et al: Metabolic heat productions, growth rate and prognosis of early breast carcinomas. In Colin, C. et al (eds.): Functional Exploration in Senology. Ghent, Belgium:European Press, 1976, pp. 93-110.
18. Hobbins, W.B. and King, B.J.: Preliminary report of thermographic

biopsy correlation. Presented at 9th Annual American Thermographic Society, Toronto, March 1979. Acta Thermograph. (In press.)

19. Aarts, N.J.: The contribution of thermography to the diagnosis of breast cancer. J. Belge Radiol. 55:71-78, 1972.

20. Amalric, R. and Spitalier, J.M.: Thermography and breast cancer. Acta Thermograph. 3:5-17, 1975.

21. Baggs, W.J. and Amor, R.L.: Thermographic screening for breast cancer in a gynecologic practice. Obstet. Gynecol. 54 (2):156-162, 1979.

22. Nyirjesy, I.: Thermography and detection of breast carcinoma. A review and comments. J. Reprod. Med. 18 (4):165-175, 1977.

23. Gautherie, M. et al: Breast thermography and cancer risk prediction. Cancer 45:51-56, 1980.

24. Byrne, R.R.: Correlation of thermography, xeromammography and biopsy in a community hospital: Preliminary report. Wis. Med. J. 73:35-37, 1974.

25. Davey, J.B., Pentney, H. et al: The early diagnosis of breast cancer. A further report for a women's screening unit. Practitioner 213:365-370, 1974.

26. Fournier, V.D.: Correlation of thermography and doubling times of breast cancer. Acta Thermograph. 3 (1-2):107-117, 1978.

27. Isard, H.J.: Breast thermography, 1980. Breast 5 (4):7-13, 1979.

28. Hobbins, W.B.: Thermography, highest risk marker in breast cancer. *In* Proceedings of Gynecological Society for the Study of Breast Disease, 1977, pp. 267-282.

29. Fisher, B., Slach, N.H. and Brosslal, I.D.J.: Cancer of the breast: Size of neoplasm and prognosis. Cancer 24:1071-1080, 1969.

30. Williams, K.L.: Thermography in the prognosis of breast cancer. Bibl. Radiol. 5:62-67, 1969.

31. Henderson, C. and Canelos, G.P.: Cancer of the breast. N. Engl. J. Med. 302:17-30, 78-90, 1980.

32. Fox, M.S.: On the diagnosis and treatment of breast cancer. JAMA 241:489-494, 1979.

Self-Evaluation Quiz

1. Blood flow in the breast is most accurately measured by:
   a) Ultrasonography
   b) Radioactive perfusion
   c) Immersion platysmography
   d) Cholesteric analysis profile
   e) Thermal monitoring

2. The first infrared thermal measurement of breast pathology in 1956 was reported by:
   a) E. Schwamm of Germany
   b) Janet Draper of England

   c) Ray Lawson of Canada
   d) Tom Love of U.S.A.

3. The circulation of the breast is basically controlled by influences on the:
   a) Parasympathetic nervous system
   b) Prolactin level
   c) Aortic pulse pressure
   c) Sympathetic nervous system

4. Anatomic development and physiologic functions both affect the observed blood flow by colorgrams.
   a) True
   b) False

5. The physiologic factors that affect colorgrams are (1) nervous system, (2) hormonal system, (3) environmental manipulation, (4) pathologic processes.
   a) True
   b) False

6. Physiologic processes such as menstruation, involution, pregnancy and lactation are bilaterally symmetrical and can be separated from pathology.
   a) True
   b) False

7. Progesterone deficiency (relative), mastopathy and mastodynia are revealed by:
   a) A wide-open vascular pattern of the entire breast
   b) Cold areas in the lateral half of the colorgram unilaterally
   c) Extremely warm nipplar/perinipplar area
   d) Hypervascular hyperthermia in the upper halves of the breast

8. The blushing or lack of blushing in one breast is usually a sign of pathology such as injury, infection, fibroadenoma or carcinoma.
   a) True
   b) False

9. Most fast-growing or "biologically significant" cancers are hot on a colorgram.
   a) True
   b) False

10. Preoperative treatment plans for breast cancer should

consider increased blood flow (abnormal colorgram) as
evidence of:

a) "Aggressive disease" in spite of stage, nodal status or
   size
b) "Limited potential disease," to be considered for lesser
   treatment protocols
c) A good autoimmune host response

11. Neo-angiogenesis in breast cancer is not under the sympa-
    thetic nervous system influence and nervous stimulation will
    not reduce blood flow in cancer cases.
    a) True
    b) False

12. It has been shown that blood flow at the time of cancer
    discovery is the best prognostic factor to date.
    a) True
    b) False

13. Thermal examination of all breast conditions with color-
    grams will add valuable information and understanding.
    a) True
    b) False

Answers on page 335.

Graphic Stress Telethermometry: An Ideal Office Screening Device for the Detection of Breast Disease

Philip G. Brooks, M.D., Alfred J. Heldfond, M.D.,
Malcolm L. Margolin, M.D., Arthur S. Allen, M.D.
and Sandi Gart, R.T.

Objectives

With the large increase in incidence of breast cancer, there is a great need for earlier diagnosis using a safe and effective screening technique. This paper will describe a computerized, infrared sensing method that functions in the office as a breast disease screening technique with these features. Included will be the results of one year's experience in 481 patients tested in a private practice setting.

Introduction

In the past several decades, breast cancer has increased dramatically in both incidence and total numbers of new cases. According to the American Cancer Society, it is estimated that 104,000 new breast cancers will be diagnosed in 1980 and that approximately one of every 11 women will develop breast cancer in her lifetime! The number of deaths from breast cancer

Philip G. Brooks, M.D., Associate Clinical Professor; Alfred J. Heldfond, M.D., Clinical Professor; Malcolm L. Margolin, M.D., Assistant Clinical Professor; Arthur S. Allen, M.D., Clinical Instructor; and Sandi Gart, R.T., Department of Obstetrics and Gynecology, University of Southern California School of Medicine and Cedars-Sinai Medical Center, Los Angeles.

Reprinted with permission, from J. Reprod. Med. 25 (1):1, 1980.

has remained virtually unchanged in the recent past, amounting to more than 30,000 deaths annually. Innovations in surgical techniques, chemotherapy and radiotherapy have made little, if any, impact on improving survival rates.

If, then, we are to make any progress in increasing the rate of survival from breast cancer, all available evidence points to early detection as the essential major thrust. One study shows that survival rates are improved by one third when the lesions are detected by a screening method, as contrasted to rates for those detected by a physician or by self-examination [1]. Another large screening study reports a significantly lower frequency of lymph node involvement when the lesion is detected by screening techniques than when detected by palpation [2].

With this as background, it is of great interest to witness the current pressure on the primary-care physician to identify the high-risk patient and to provide careful monitoring and screening procedures for early detection of breast disease. The American College of Obstetricians and Gynecologists, for example, in a statement of policy, recommends annual mammographic screening for all women over age 50, for those 35 to 50 as a baseline, and for those in whom high-risk factors exist [3].

Despite its diagnostic accuracy, x-ray mammography does not fulfill the requirements of an ideal screening tool. To begin with, there are insufficient competent radiographers to reach the entire at-risk female population. Furthermore, 25% of all breast cancers occur in women under age 50. Patients and their physicians are very reticent to begin mammographic screening at age 35 or younger because of the fear of the cumulative hazard from repeated examination [4].

The ideal screening device should be one that can be employed in the primary-care office or clinic. It must be safe, inexpensive and cost-effective, reasonably accurate in delineating high-risk and low-risk subpopulations, and simple enough for the primary-care physician to interpret. This paper will report on a new office device that may fulfill these requirements.

Instrumentation

Graphic stress telethermometry (GST) (Fig. 1) is a direct, noninvasive, heat-sensing technique that utilizes a micro-

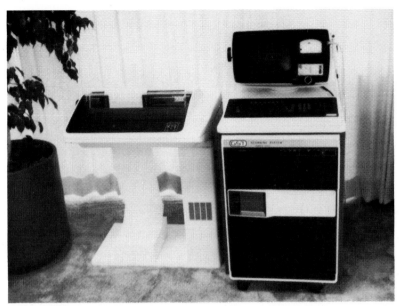

FIG. 1. Graphic stress telethermometry unit: microprocessor and printer.

processor to record precise temperature measurements. The sensing unit is a thermopile infrared sensor (Figs. 2 and 3), which when hand-held from a distance of 1 to 2 cm from the skin over the breast, very accurately measures the temperature of that portion of the breast. The computer is programmed to analyze the recorded temperatures and to detect areas of abnormal thermal activity. A three-page report is generated from an attached printer immediately after completion of the evaluation. In addition to the recorded historical and identifying information, the report includes all recorded temperatures, a histogram depicting the patterns of heat emission and a simplified map of each breast wherein the computer has marked the areas of concern. The computer assesses a score, from 1 through 99, which relates to the relative risk of there being suspicious breast pathology, based on experience accumulated from a large data base of normal and pathologic examinations. Factors that adversely affect the GST score include asymmetrical temperatures of each breast (contralateral and ipsilateral asymmetry), abnormal cooling responses and relationships to forehead and nipple thermal activity. Menstrual timing of the examination has little effect on the score, although, for

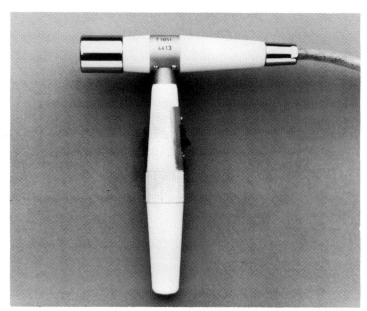

FIG. 2. Thermopile sensor: hand-held infrared sensing wand.

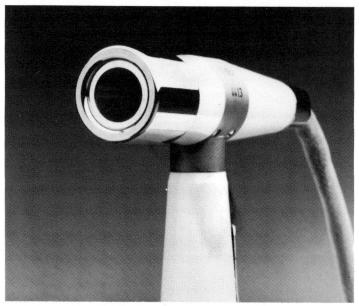

FIG. 3. Close-up of sensor head.

standardization, most of these tests were done in the post-menstrual phase of the cycle. Serial tests show excellent reproducibility irrespective of change in technicians.

Procedure

After filling out a single-page questionnaire regarding symptoms and history, the patient lies supine in the examination room with the breasts uncovered for five to ten minutes. The ambient temperature of the room should be maintained at 20° to 23° C. for ideal equilibration, and strong drafts should be avoided. After the technician processes the historical and identifying data, the computer displays the steps to be followed in scanning the breasts. The sensor is passed over eight sectors of each breast slowly and in a prescribed sequence. Nipple and forehead temperatures are recorded also for comparison. The entire procedure is then repeated immediately following immersion of the patient's hands in ice water for 15 seconds. This stress results in the regular cooling of normal breasts and forehead of from 0.3° to 1.0° C. Lesions with increased metabolism, such as carcinoma, fibrocystic disease and some fibroadenomas, show decreased cooling patterns. The unique features of this technique, in contrast to other screening methods, include (1) direct infrared sensing without dependence on photographic film, lenses and differential nipple or chest wall focusing; (2) testing in the supine position to eliminate "blind" areas in large breasts; and (3) use of ice stress to minimize surface vascular thermal contributions.

Study Method

In the year between September 1, 1978 and August 31, 1979, 481 patients underwent GST screening in our private office. No patient had palpable masses, nipple discharge or other acute symptoms. Our indications for recommending GST were age of 35 or over, family history of breast cancer, and a prior history of breast problems (excluding the young patient with so-called fibrocystic breast disease symptoms or palpatory findings).

GST scores from 1 through 40 were grouped as class 1, believed to be at low risk; from 41 through 80, class 2, or intermediate risk; and from 81 through 99, class 3 or high risk. X-ray mammography was ordered for any patient whose GST score or pattern was suggestive of a pathologic lesion. Referral to a breast surgeon for consultation and/or biopsy followed, as indicated.

Results

The distribution of scores is listed in Table 1, and is compared with the distribution of scores in an assumed random, unselected population of asymptomatic women.

Table 2 lists the frequency with which patients expressed positive breast symptomatology in the above-mentioned questionnaire. Also listed are percentages of breast symptoms reported in a random sampling of women and in biopsy-proven breast cancer patients [5].

Table 3 lists the follow-up data and results of our first year's experience with the GST system for office screening. If breast cancers picked up or missed are endpoints in the evaluation of a new breast screening device, then our numbers are too small and the follow-up period too short to be statistically significant.

Discussion

Initial validation of the efficacy of the GST system was reported by Snyder [5]. In a study of 315 biopsy-proven patients, only 7% of cancers fell into the low-risk (or class 1) category. Almost two thirds of the cancers fell into the high-risk group. In addition, she reported that the size of the lesion had no effect on the scores or the frequency of false-negatives.

Table 1. Distribution of GST Scores

GST Score	Private Practice No.	%	Assumed Normal Population %
1-40 (class 1)	209	43	65
41-80 (class 2)	221	46	30
81-99 (class 3)	51	11	5
Total	481	100	100

Table 2. Patients Reporting Symptoms

	No.	%
Private practice	221	46
Normal population	–	18
Breast cancer patients	59	95

In our study, it can be noted that a higher percentage of patients had intermediate and high-risk scores than that seen in a random sampling of women. This result reflects selection of patients with known risk factors. The implication is that those patients most interested in and accepting of new modalities are those who, because of breast symptoms or family history, are more likely to have fibrocystic breasts (and higher scores) and are more frightened of breast disease.

While only one cancer was detected, the four other biopsies showed "severe mammary dysplasia." Is this a premalignant lesion in the breast as it is in the cervix? Only long-term monitoring and careful follow-up will determine the risks in these patients. It is our belief that the serial reproducibility of GST and the permanent, objective patterns displayed on the histogram allow close monitoring which is far better and safer than that of any previous technique.

It should be noted that in the case of the one carcinoma detected, the mammogram was negative and the ultimate biopsy was performed six months after the initially suspicious GST, as a result of the development of a bloody nipple discharge.

Table 3. Results of Screening

X-ray mammography ordered – 23

GST class 1 – 0
GST class 2 – 14
GST class 3 – 9

Patients biopsied – 5

GST class 1 – 0
GST class 2 – 3*
GST class 3 – 2†

*Pathologic diagnoses: severe mammary dysplasia, 3.
†Pathologic diagnoses: severe mammary dysplasia, 1; intraductal carcinoma, 1.

Finally, the benefit of the GST system as a negative examination also should be reported. Several of our patients had breasts that were difficult to examine accurately because of diffuse granularity. X-ray mammography showed no lesions suspicious for carcinoma, but the fear of false radiographic negativity, reported to be higher for this type of breasts, was lessened by discovering benign-appearing GST patterns.

At present we are working with the company that manufactures the device in La Jolla, California, to add more parameters and data to the current data base of approximately 12,000 patients. As more nationwide testing results are accumulated, we expect to approach our goal of 75% of all scores in class 1, 20% in class 2, and 5% in class 3, with virtually all highly suspicious lesions falling into the upper risk categories.

Conclusions

Although there is no current nonsurgical procedure that is 100% accurate in detecting early breast cancer, the GST system is a highly effective, direct heat-measuring, screening test. It is noninvasive, highly suitable for office screening and harmless. There were no false-negatives in our study. The ice-stress procedure minimizes false-positives. The computerized objective analysis and risk assessment make the procedure relatively simple and quick for clinicians to use in their practices. Finally, the reproducibility and objective graphic printouts allow for frequent monitoring, with the ability to compare the patterns to denote improvement or deterioration of suspicious areas.

References

1. Shapiro, S., Strax, P., Venet, L. et al: Changes in 5-year breast cancer mortality in a breast cancer screening program. *In* Proceedings of the Seventh National Cancer Conference. New York:American Cancer Society and National Cancer Institute, 1972, pp. 663-687.
2. Hicks, M.J., Davis, J.R., Layton, J.M. and Present, A.J.: Sensitivity of mammography and physical examination of the breast for detecting breast cancer. JAMA 242:2080-2083, 1979.
3. Statement of Policy on Mammography. American College of Obstetrics and Gynecology, Sept. 1979.
4. Upton, A.C.: Report of NCI working group on the risks associated with mammography in mass screening for detection of breast cancer. Bethesda:National Cancer Institute, 1977.

5. Synder, R., Watson, R.C. and Cruz, N.: Graphic stress telether-mometry: A possible supplement to physical examination in screening for abnormalities in the female breast. Am. J. Diag. Gynecol. Obstet. 1:197, 1979.

Self-Evaluation Quiz

1. There is no evidence that breast cancer survival is improved when the lesions are detected by screening techniques, in contrast to those detected by palpation.
   a) True
   b) False

2. The technique of graphic stress telethermometry en-compasses all of the following *except*:
   a) Computer recording and analysis of the data
   b) Repeating the test procedure after immersing the patient's hands in ice water, to minimize false-positives
   c) A small but acceptable x-ray dosage
   d) An immediate printed report of the results

3. The GST system is designed to provide an office procedure as opposed to being limited to major institutions.
   a) True
   b) False

4. The computerized report generated from a GST examina-tion lists all the following categories *except*:
   a) Low risk
   b) Intermediate risk
   c) High risk
   d) Definite cancer

5. With the GST system, the patient is tested in the upright position.
   a) True
   b) False

6. In a study of biopsy-proven cancers, how many showed high-risk GST scores?
   a) All
   b) One third
   c) Two thirds

Answers on page 335.

Physiology and Pathology
of Breast Disease

The Significance of Nipple Discharge

Henry Patrick Leis, Jr., M.D.

Objectives

The purpose of this paper is to provide the reader a knowledge of the following:

1. The frequency of nipple discharge in benign and malignant breast lesions, and which types are of significance.
2. The classification and epidemiology of various types of nipple discharges.
3. The frequency of association of various types. of discharges with cancer and factors that increase the risk of cancer association.
4. The medical and surgical management of patients with nipple discharges.

Frequency

Nipple discharge is a relatively common symptom in patients with breast disease [1-6]. In a series of 7,588 breast operations from New York Medical College between 1950 and 1977, the chief complaint in 6,450 patients (85%) was a lump and the second most common complaint was a nipple discharge, occurring in 560 patients (7.4%). In the office and clinic it is an even more common complaint since many patients with nipple discharge can be treated medically and do not require surgery.

Henry Patrick Leis, Jr., M.D., F.A.C.S., F.I.C.S. (Hon.), Clinical Professor of Surgery, Chief of Breast Service; Co-Director, Institute of Breast Diseases, New York Medical College, Valhalla, N.Y.; Chief of Breast Surgery, Cabrini Medical Center, New York City.

Significant Discharges

To be of significance a discharge should be true, spontaneous and persistent and, of course, nonlactational. True discharges come through a mammary duct or ducts and appear on the surface of the nipple. Secretions or exudates can occur in patients with inverted nipples, eczematoid lesions, traumatic erosions, herpes simplex, Montgomery gland infections and mammary duct fistulae, resulting in the appearance of a pseudodischarge of varied color and consistency on or near the surface of the nipple that can mimic a true discharge.

With the increasing popularity of self-examinations and of periodic breast examinations by physicians, more and more women and doctors are discovering that firm squeezing of the nipple and subareolar area may result in the expression of a drop or two of cloudy, milky, gray or green, thick fluid. This is especially true if they are taking oral contraceptives, tranquilizers or rauwolfia alkaloids, if they have been recently castrated or if they are perimenopausal. These patients should be reassured that this does not indicate a pathologic condition.

We feel that to be of significance a nipple discharge should be spontaneous and persistent. Sartorius [7], however, has reported that the cytologic study of nonspontaneous discharges obtained from asymptomatic women by the use of a small suction kit, called a Breast Pap Kit, can be rewarding. He stated that he had obtained secretions in 72% of asymptomatic women and that occasionally cytologic examination revealed an underlying cancer without any other findings. It must be emphasized that his results have been hard to duplicate in other centers and that the number of cancers that might be detected with this technique would be extremely small.

Classification

Classification into one of the seven basic types of nipple discharge — i.e. milky, multicolored and sticky, purulent, clear or watery, yellow or serous, pink or serosanquineous, and bloody or sanguineous — is usually quite easy by observing the color and consistency of the discharge, by feeling it to see if it is sticky and by staining a slide of it with Wright's stain to see whether pus or blood is present.

Sometimes discharges due to duct ectasia can appear bloody but are not. A simple test in the office to determine the presence or absence of blood is to test the discharge with a Hemostix or to put it on a white sponge. If blood is present a red color will appear, with lighter shadings of red extending to the periphery, but this will not be the case in discharges that appear bloody but are not.

Etiology

Nipple discharge is more common in patients with benign rather than malignant lesions. In our 560 patients operated on for nipple discharge, the discharge occurred in 493 out of 5,424 patients with benign lesions (or 9.1%) and in 67 out of 2,164 patients with cancers (or 3.1%). Among males it had a more serious prognostic import [8], occurring in 4 out of 20 patients with cancer (or 20%) [4].

Cancer Association

The importance of nipple discharge rests in its frequency of association with cancer, with the reported incidence in the literature ranging from 3% to 47% [9]. The types of discharge associated with cancer are the watery, serous, serosanguineous and bloody.

Of our 503 patients operated on for one of these types of discharges, 67 (13.3%) had cancers, 36 (7.2%) had marked atypias designated as precancerous mastopathies [10] and 60 (11.9%) had mild to moderate atypical changes; 163 patients (32.4%) had either cancers or atypias [4]. Seltzer et al [11] reported a 23% incidence of associated cancers and McLaughlin [9] reported 26%, but no reference was made to precancerous mastopathies.

There is an increasing incidence of associated cancers when the discharge is accompanied by a lump; when it is of a certain type — with the order of increasing frequency being serous, serosanguineous, bloody and the rare watery; when it is unilateral and from a single duct; when there are adverse cytologic and breast x-ray findings; and when it occurs in patients over 50 years of age [4].

Palpable Mass

In the papillomatosis type of fibrocystic disease and in intraductal papillomas, it is common not to be able to palpate a mass. This is unusual when cancer is the etiologic factor, but it can occur. There was no palpable mass in 8 of our 67 patients with cancers (11.9%) or in 16 of 78 patients with cancers (20.5%) reported by Seltzer et al [11].

Discharges Associated with Cancers

Milky, multicolored and sticky, purulent discharges are rarely if ever associated with cancers but the serous, sero-sanguineous, bloody and rare watery types are. As to the frequency of these various types of surgically significant discharges in our 503 patients, 11 (2.2%) were watery, 207 (41.1%) were serous, 160 (31.8%) were serosanguineous and 125 (24.9%) were bloody.

Cancers were associated in 13 of the 207 patients with serous discharges (or 6.3%), in 19 of the 160 serosanguineous discharges (or 11.9%), in 30 of the 125 with bloody discharges (or 24.0%) and in 5 of the 11 patients with watery discharges (or 45.4%). From this it can be seen that the watery discharge, while rare, must be regarded with concern [4].

Most of these types of discharge occurred in patients with benign lesions. Among the 503 patients the discharges were due to intraductal papillomas in 231 (45.9%), to fibrocystic disease in 181 (36.9%), to advanced duct ectasia in 24 (4.8%) and to cancer in 67 (13.3%). As previously mentioned, another 96 patients (19.1%), especially those with intraductal papillomas or the papillomatosis type of fibrocystic disease, had mild to marked atypical changes. These discharges, especially the bloody type, were also seen in patients with near-term pregnancies and were due to vascular engorgement, but none of these patients underwent operation.

Unilateral and Single-Duct Discharges

In the relationship to cancer and precancerous mastopathy, unilateral and single-duct discharges are the most important [12]. A watery, serous, serosanguineous or bloody unilateral, single-duct discharge is usually due to an intraductal papilloma or cancer.

Milky and multicolored sticky discharges are commonly bilateral and from multiple ducts; they represent benign entities. Purulent discharges are usually unilateral and from more than one duct, but these are easily recognized by their associated underlying infection. Despite the importance of unilaterality and single-duct discharge, one can not ignore bilateral and multiple-duct discharges if they are of the watery, serous, serosanguineous or bloody type. While uncommon, intraductal papillomas and cancers can be bilateral; the papillomatosis of fibrocystic disease, which is associated with a considerable percentage of precancerous mastopathies, is frequently bilateral, although it usually presents as discharge from multiple ducts. About 14% to 20% of intraductal papillomas are multiple; discharges due to these lesions may be elicited from more than one duct. Even cancer can involve more than one duct, with resulting multiple-duct discharge.

Cytologic Examination

Cytologic examination should be a routine part of the examination of every patient with a nipple discharge. Its reliability depends on the diligence and training of the cytologist and on the technique of preparing the smear [13]. As with other diagnostic aids, one must recognize its limitations but not disregard its advantages. One must not rely on cytology as an absolute means of establishing whether a discharge is due to a benign or malignant lesion, since there is a relatively high percentage of false-negatives and of atypical changes, and even an occasional false-positive.

In our series of 560 patients operated on for nipple discharge, 11 (16.4%) of the 67 patients with cancers had false-negative results. Of the remaining 493 patients with benign lesions, 91 (18.5%) had mild to marked atypical changes and 10 (2%) had false-positive results [4].

Breast X-rays

Breast x-rays (mammography or xerography) offer an additional aid in localizing and diagnosing the etiologic factor in nipple discharge. It must be remembered, however, that a negative breast x-ray does not mean that there could not be a cancer, and biopsy must never be deferred because of this. Seven of our 67 patients with cancers (or 10.4%) had negative x-ray findings.

Soft tissue x-rays are the ones that are commonly used. Their accuracy in determining whether there is an underlying malignancy is quite good, but their accuracy in visualizing and localizing small intraductal papillomas is not good. Because of this, Funderbunk and Syphax [14] and others [15] have emphasized the importance of using contrast mammography in patients with a nipple discharge but no palpable mass.

Patient's Age

The patient's age is an important factor in evaluating the etiologic basis of a nipple discharge. Milky discharges usually are seen in the childbearing years. Multicolored sticky discharges have a common age range of 37 to 58, with a median age of 43. Purulent discharges can occur at any age, but they are commonly associated with patients in the childbearing years.

Of our 503 patients with the surgically significant discharges, i.e. watery, serous, serosanguineous and bloody, the youngest patient was 13 and the oldest was 94; most discharges occurred in the fourth decade. Eight (1.6%) were under 20, 70 (13.9%) were between 20 and 29, 176 (35.0%) were between 30 and 39, 145 (28.9%) were between 40 and 49, and 104 (20.6%) were over 50 [4].

The median age for patients with one of these discharges due to an intraductal papilloma was 40. It was 34 for those with fibrocystic disease, 43 for those with duct ectasia and 56 for those with cancers. After the age of 50, cancer becomes an increasingly common cause. Of our 104 patients over the age of 50 with one of these discharges, 53 had cancers (or 50.9%) [4]. McLaughlin [9] reported that nipple discharge was associated with an underlying malignancy in 64% of patients over 50, and Robbins [16] reported that more than 50% of women with one of these discharges over the age of 60 had an associated cancer.

Treatment

The treatment of patients with nipple discharge depends on the type and etiology of the discharge, and it can be either medical or surgical.

Medical Treatment

Galactorrhea results in the production of bilateral, multiple-duct, spontaneous, milky discharge. It is thought to be due to an increase in the production of prolactin either by direct action in the pituitary gland or by removing it from hypothalamic inhibition. It can occur in patients with normal ovulatory function and is most often seen following pregnancy, lasting one or more years. It also occurs in patients with endocrine disorders that are associated with amenorrhea, such as the Chiari-Frommel, Forbes-Albright and Del Castillo syndromes. Some drugs, such as the phenothiazines, tricyclic antidepressants, rauwolfia alkaloids and methyldopa, can cause it. Oral contraceptives seem to produce this type of discharge more commonly when there is associated amenorrhea. Pituitary adenomas are now recognized as a not uncommon cause.

Treatment is basically medical unless there is a pituitary adenoma which must be removed surgically. It is directed toward removing the cause whenever possible and toward reducing prolactin production by the administration of large doses of estrogen, toward inhibiting prolactin production by giving progesterone or toward stimulating the hypothalamus by administering clomiphene.

Duct ectasia or comedomastitis can produce a multicolored, sticky, spontaneous, multiple-duct, commonly bilateral discharge. Surgery is not indicated unless there is a mass or the discharge changes to a serous, serosanguineous or bloody type. The patient is advised to wash both nipples gently with cotton pledgets soaked in pHisoHex or Betadine scrub for two to five minutes daily and to avoid nipple manipulation. Occasionally, estrogen therapy can be helpful in older patients.

Patients with acute puerperal mastitis, chronic lactational mastitis, central breast abscess or advanced duct ectasia (plasma cell mastitis) can have a purulent discharge through one or more ducts. While some patients respond to appropriate antibiotic therapy, suppuration and abscess formation require incision and drainage. In addition to taking smears and preparing cultures for the predominant organism and antibiotic sensitivity tests, a portion of the abscess wall should be removed for histologic study to be sure that there is no underlying cancer with secondary necrosis and infection.

Surgical Treatment

We feel that surgical exploration [17] is mandatory in patients with watery, serous, serosanguineous or bloody discharge, since these are associated with a sizable percentage of cancers and precancerous mastopathies, and since cancer can be the etiologic factor despite negative cytology (16.4%) or negative x-ray findings (10.4%) and without a palpable mass (11.9%). The exception is a patient with a near-term pregnancy who does not have a palpable mass or positive cytology. Usually the discharge clears up within a few weeks after delivery when the vascular engorgement subsides. If it persists, then surgical exploration is recommended.

Surgical Technique

In women under 30 or in those anxious to have children, only the clinically involved duct, which usually is easily detected by its size and bluish color, is excised with a surrounding wedge of breast tissue. In the remaining patients we advise a complete excision of the central ducts to ensure removal of all papillomas, all the diffuse changes found in papillomatosis and all the central tissue that might harbor a small in situ carcinoma [18-20].

Surgical exploration can be done through a nipple-splitting or a circumareolar-type incision. We prefer the latter because we feel that it offers better cosmetic results. We have not found it necessary or desirable to probe the affected duct with a fine lacrimal probe or blunted needle, as is sometimes advised.

The central point of the circumareolar incision is placed over a mass if one is present or, if not, over the pressure point area that produces the discharge. The incision is never carried more than halfway around the areola, to ensure good blood supply.

The incision is carried down through the subcutanous tissue and then an areolar flap is developed, using sharp dissection and skin hooks for traction. The dissection is carried up to the central terminal ducts which can be seen going up into the nipple.

The central terminal ducts are dissected free on each side and encircled with a clamp. The ducts are then tied to prevent loss of their contents, to serve as a marker for the pathologist and to help with traction.

The nipple is coned out, transecting the ducts flush with the skin to ensure their complete removal. This is best accomplished by the surgeon using his index finger to invert the nipple during the sharp dissection.

When the nipple and areola have been completely elevated, a diamond-shaped incision is made around the central ducts. We prefer this type of incision to a circular one because it allows for a better closure of the deep tissues.

Then the incision is carried deep into the breast parenchyma, beyond any clinical evidence of dilated ducts or adverse findings, and the central ducts are removed.

After careful hemostasis is established, a detailed repair with interrupted 00 chromic catgut sutures is done in line with the circumareolar incision.

The nipple and areola are placed back in position without any tacking sutures, since these are prone to produce dimpling, and the circumareolar incision is then closed with fine, interrupted nonabsorbable Stewart sutures to prevent inversion of the edges.

We rely on pressure dressings with a central cut-out for the nipple rather than using drainage. The nipple has openings where the discharge was coming from and these usually will serve as drainage areas, although sometimes aspiration is necessary. A dressing without the central cut-out can obstruct this drainage and also result in nipple retraction.

The cosmetic results with this technique are usually quite satisfactory, as can be seen by examining the appearance of the incision and of the nipple and areola after only four weeks and again after six months, when the incision is often difficult to see.

Unless there is an obvious cancer it may be better to rely on permanent paraffin sections rather than on frozen sections, since it can be quite difficult to differentiate premalignant lesions from in situ carcinomas. There is no statistically valid evidence to indicate that a delay of five to seven days between biopsy and definitive therapy influences the survival of the patient [17].

Summary

Nipple discharge is an important clinical entity, being the chief complaint in 560 (7.4%) of 7,588 patients undergoing breast surgery at New York Medical College between 1950 and 1977.

Most of the seven basic types — i.e. milky, multicolored and sticky, purulent, clear or watery, yellow or serous, pink or serosanguineous, and bloody or sanguineous — are due to benign lesions. However, in 503 patients with one of the last four types of discharge, 67 (13.3%) had cancers, 36 (7.2%) had precancerous mastopathies and 60 (11.9%) had mild to moderate atypical changes. Surgical exploration is mandatory in patients with one of these types of discharge, since they can be due to a cancer without a palpable mass and with a negative cytology and x-ray.

There is an increasing incidence of assorted cancers when the discharge is accompanied by a lump; when it is, in order of increasing frequency, a serous, serosanguineous, bloody or watery type; when it is unilateral and from a single duct; when there are adverse cytologic and x-ray changes; and when the patient is over 50 years of age.

References

1. Leis, H.P., Jr.: Diagnosis and Treatment of Breast Lesions. Flushing, N.Y.:Medical Examination Publishing Co., 1970, p. 91.
2. Leis, H.P., Jr.: Evaluation of nipple discharge. In Gallagher, H.S. (ed.): Early Breast Cancer Detection and Treatment. New York:John Wiley and Sons, Inc., 1975, p. 69.
3. Leis, H.P., Jr.: The diagnosis of breast cancer. CA 27:209, 1977.
4. Leis, H.P., Jr. and Cammarata, A.: Nipple discharge: Evaluation, cancer association and management. Am. J. Diag. Gynecol. Obstet. 1:43, 1979.

5. Leis, H.P., Jr., Pilnik, S. and Cammarata, A.: Diagnosis of nipple discharge. Female Patient 1:22, 1976.
6. Pilnik, S. and Leis, H.P., Jr.: Nipple discharge. *In* Gallagher, H.S., Leis, H.P., Jr., Snyderman, R.K. and Urban, J.A. (eds.): The Breast. St. Louis:C. V. Mosby Co., 1978, p. 524.
7. Sartorius, O.W.: Breast duct cytology. Presented at Thirteenth Annual Conference on Detection and Treatment of Early Breast Cancer, American College of Radiologists, Orlando, Fla., 1974.
8. Holleb, A.I. and Farrow, J.H.: The significance of nipple discharge. CA 16:182, 1966.
9. McLaughlin, C.W., Jr.: Nipple discharge. Mod. Med. 43:57, 1975.
10. Leis, H.P., Jr., Urban, J.A. and Snyderman, R.K.: Management of potentially malignant lesions. *In* Gallager, H.S., Leis, H.P., Jr., Snyderman, R.K. and Urban, J.A. (eds.): The Breast. St. Louis:C. V. Mosby Co., 1978, p. 208.
11. Seltzer, M.H., Perloff, L.J., Kelley, R.I. and Fitts, W.T., Jr.: The significance of age in patients with nipple discharge. Surg. Gynecol. Obstet. 70:519, 1970.
12. Rosemond, G.P. and Maier, W.P.: Nonlactational nipple discharge. J. Dis. Breast 1:23, 1975.
13. Christopherson, W.M.: Present role of cytology in cancer detection and diagnosis. Cancer 18:29, 1968.
14. Funderburk, W.W. and Syphax, B.: Evaluation of nipple discharge in benign and malignant diseases. Cancer 24:1290, 1969.
15. Bjorn-Hansen, R.: Contrast mammography. Br. J. Radiol. 38:947, 1965.
16. Robbins, G.F.: Nipple discharge. Mod. Med. 43:57, 1975.
17. Cammarata, A., Rosen, P.P. and Leis, H.P., Jr.: Breast biopsy: Surgical aspects, role of frozen sections and specimen radiography. *In* Gallager, H.S., Leis, H.P., Jr., Snyderman, R.K. and Urban, J.A. (eds.): The Breast. St. Louis:C. V. Mosby Co., 1978, p. 155.
18. Leis, H.P., Jr. and Pilnik, S.: Nipple discharge. Hosp. Med. 6:29, 1970.
19. Leis, H.P., Jr.: Selective and reconstructive surgical procedures for carcinoma of the breast. Surg. Gynecol. Obstet. 148:27, 1979.
20. Leis, H.P., Jr.: Selective moderate surgical approach for potentially curable breast cancer. *In* Gallager, H.S., Leis, H.P., Jr., Snyderman, R.K. and Urban, J.A. (eds.): The Breast. St. Louis:C. V. Mosby Co., 1978, p. 232.

Self-Evaluation Quiz

1. After a lump, nipple discharge is the next most common complaint of patients admitted to the hospital for breast surgery.
   a) True
   b) False

2. Nipple discharge is of significance except in which one of the following?
   a) When it is true
   b) When it is spontaneous
   c) When it is nonlactational
   d) When it is bilateral
3. Nipple discharge is more likely to be associated with cancer except in which one of the following?
   a) When it is associated with a lump
   b) When it comes through multiple ducts
   c) When it is unilateral
   d) When it occurs in patients over 50 years of age
4. The following types of nipple discharge, in order of increasing frequency, can be associated with cancer: serous, serosanguineous, bloody and watery.
   a) True
   b) False
5. A unilateral, single-duct, serous, serosanguineous, bloody or watery type of nipple discharge can be associated with a cancer even if there is no palpable mass and the cytology and mammogram are negative.
   a) True
   b) False
6. Cytologic examination of a nipple discharge must not be relied upon to differentiate benign from malignant lesions because there is a relatively high percentage of false-negatives.
   a) True
   b) False
7. Galactorrhea can occur in patients with normal ovulatory function and is most often seen for one or more years following pregnancy.
   a) True
   b) False
8. A multicolored, bilateral, sticky discharge, without a palpable mass, can usually be treated medically and does not require surgery.
   a) True
   b) False

9. In women under 30 and in those anxious to have children, with a bloody, single-duct, unilateral discharge, complete excision of the central ducts is not advised, but only excision of the involved duct with a surrounding wedge of breast tissue.
   a) True
   b) False

10. When there is no palpable mass, the central point of the circumareolar incision for central duct excision is placed over the pressure point that produces the discharge.
    a) True
    b) False

Answers on page 335.

The Endocrine Physiology of the Breast

Abraham E. Rakoff, M.D.

Objective

The purpose of this paper is to review the present status of the hormonal regulation of the breast, with particular reference to those hormones which are involved in growth and development, and those involved in lactation.

The mammary gland is a hormone-responsive organ, the endocrine control of which involves many hormones and hormone receptors. Indeed, all of the endocrine glands are concerned to a greater or lesser degree in its growth, development and functions, including the ovary, the hypothalamus, the adenohypophysis, the neurohypophysis, the adrenals, the pancreas, the thyroid, the parathyroids and the placenta. There is now a voluminous literature dealing with experimental and clinical observations on the effect of hormones on the mammary glands and lactation. In this brief review it is not feasible to cite individual references. Several pertinent reviews are listed in the bibliography.

Hormones Influencing Mammary Growth and Development

Although early fetal differentiation and growth of the mammary buds is not dependent on hormonal influences, fetal breast tissue becomes increasingly responsive to hormones, particularly the placental hormones, as gestation progresses.

Abraham E. Rakoff, M.D., Emeritus Professor of Obstetrics and Gynecology, Honorary Professor of Medicine (Endocrinology), Jefferson Medical College, Thomas Jefferson University, Philadelphia, Pa.

This is clinically evident by the stimulated state of the mammary discs which may be observed in neonates of both sexes, as well as the presence of secretion ("witch's milk") in some instances. The effect of testicular hormone in the male fetus leads to significant changes in the differentiation of the rudimentary breast into male and female types. Although some growth of breast tissue occurs during infancy, proportional to body growth (isometric), an active or allometric spurt occurs in the prepubertal phase and appears to be clearly related to increasing ovarian function.

Estrogen and Progesterone

The prepubertal spurt in breast development, which in the human female begins between the ages of 9 and 11, and its subsequent development are initiated primarily by estrogen. It begins with enlargement in the size of the nipple, an increase in size of the areola and then proliferation of the duct system. As the ovarian estrogen secretion rises, the ducts increase in length and thickness and small knobs appear at the distal ends of the tubules which will later form the acini under the combined stimulation of progesterone and estrogen. It is quite evident from numerous observations that progesterone is necessary for maximal alveolar development.

Women are well aware of cyclic changes in the size, structure and degree of tenderness of their breasts during the menstrual cycle. These are correlated with the rise and fall in estrogen and progesterone during the ovulatory cycle, and are accompanied by histologic and histochemical changes. During the proliferative phase of the cycle, the rising titer of estrogens induces parenchymal proliferation, increased cellular RNA synthesis and associated nuclear changes. With the rise of progesterone during the luteal phase of the cycle, the mammary ducts become somewhat dilated, the alveolar cells differentiate into secretory cells, and some lipid droplets appear which may show signs of secretion into the alveolar lumen. During the premenstrual phase, there is an increase in breast volume due to lobular edema, infiltration of perilobular mammary stroma with fluids, lymphoid and plasma cells, enlargement of alveolar luminal diameters and appearance of intra-alveolar secretory material. During menstruation, there is some mammary secretion associated with the withdrawal of the luteal sex steroids. During the postmenstrual phase regressive changes occur, including reduction in lobular-alveolar size, narrowing of alveolar lumina, decrease in tissue edema and degeneration and necrosis of some glandular cells. The breasts decrease to their smallest size from about days 4 to 7 of the cycle.

The remarkable increase in ductular-lobular-alveolar growth that occurs during pregnancy is attributable to an increase in estrogen and progesterone secreted by the corpus luteum and placenta, as well as prolactin, placental lactogen and chorionic gonadotropin. The progressive histologic changes that occur during gestation include sprouting of terminal ductal tubules, replacement of mammary fat tissue by glandular tissue, secretory changes in the alveolar epithetium and accumulation of secretional products in the alveolar lumina with enhanced secretion of colostrum.

With failing ovarian function after the menopause, there is a progressive reduction in glandular tissue, an increase in fat deposition and a relative predominance of connective tissue.

Although estrogen is the prime hormone in stimulating mammary growth at puberty, and estrogen and progesterone are chiefly responsible for further development during the normal menstrual cycle, hormones other than those secreted by the ovary appear to play a significant role (Fig. 1). Thus, for example, although the breasts tend to become smaller following bilateral oophorectomy, some degree of stimulation of mammary tissue may continue if the other endocrine glands, particular the pituitary, the adrenals and the thyroid, are intact. Isometric growth of the breasts may continue if castration is performed during the prepubertal phase. It has also been shown in rodents that mammary development is not observed following castration unless the animals are, in addition, adrenalectomized or hypophysectomized. Such observations have led to the now widely held opinion that the ovary plays an important, but not exclusive, role in mammary growth.

The overriding influence of estrogen and progesterone in breast development is noted particularly in patients who have been ovarian deficient from prepuberty on. For example, in patients with typical Turner syndrome, breast development does not occur until estrogen is added, following which the

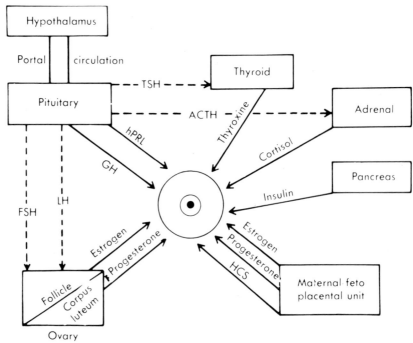

FIG. 1. Endocrine factors influencing breast development and function.
FSH, follicle-stimulating hormone; LH, luteinizing hormone; TSH, thy-
roid-stimulating hormone; hPRL, prolactin; GH, growth hormone; HCS,
human chorionic somatomammotropin (human placental lactogen). (From
Reyniak, J.V.: Physiology of the breast. *In* Gallager, H.S., Leis, H.P., Jr.,
Snyderman, R.K. and Urban, J.A. (eds.): The Breast. St. Louis:C. V.
Mosby Co., 1978, pp. 23-32.)

nipples, areola and glandular tissue, chiefly ductal, develop
(Tanner class 3); full development with acinar tissue (Tanner
class 5) may be induced by substitutional therapy with cyclic
estrogen and progesterone administration.

The responsiveness of the breast to hormones which
stimulate its growth is apparently influenced by genetic factors,
although the mechanisms by which they operate are not known.
Thus, for example, in normal women with apparently identical
hormonal patterns, the degree of breast development may vary
greatly from those with very small breasts to those who are
abundantly endowed, and even to those with markedly excessive growth of breast tissue. Even in the same individual,

marked difference in development of one breast compared with the other is not uncommon, and in some instances is so great as to be bizarre. In otherwise normal women who are unhappy because of the small size of their breasts, the administration of hormones has little, if any, lasting effect in increasing their size, although high doses of estrogens, especially diethylstilbestrol, may increase the size and darken the nipples and areola. The administration to normal females of estrogen and progestins, as in oral contraceptives, may temporarily increase the fullness of the breasts by stimulating acinar growth and stromal edema, but this generally regresses to pretreatment status when the pills are discontinued.

Much the same is true of the patient with marked enlargement of the breasts, including those with enormous adolescent or virginal hypertrophy. Endocrine studies consistently fail to reveal an excess of estrogen, progesterone, prolactin or other hormones. Indeed, some of these patients may actually become amenorrheic and estrogen-deficient as the result of the psychic stress associated with their breast problems, but without significant effect on breast size.

Another interesting interplay of the influence of genetic and endocrine factors in breast development is seen in patients with the feminizing testicular syndrome. These patients, who are phenotypic females with very well-developed breasts despite the presence of testes, have a genetic defect in that the male target organs are nonresponsive to androgen; in utero they fail to develop accessory male genital structures and as adults they do not develop pubic or axillary hair. Their breast tissue, however, is highly responsive to estrogen, presumably of testicular and adrenal origin, possibly because of the lack of an androgen influence during fetal development.

Anterior Pituitary

The mammary gland response to the administration of estrogen and progesterone in oophorectomized-hypophysectomized animals is blunted as compared to nonhypophysectomized castrates. The inadequate response can be overcome by the addition of pituitary extracts. It was such observations which led to the belief that the pituitary secreted "mammogenic" hormones. It is now generally accepted that these mammogenic pituitary hormones are prolactin and growth hormone, both of which appear to augment the action of estrogen and progesterone on the breasts.

Although the role of prolactin in mammary growth is not fully known, there is increasing evidence that prolactin is an important growth-stimulatory hormone and plays a significant role in regulating the response of the breast to estrogen and progesterone.

Another pituitary hormone that also may have an indirect augmentation action is ACTH, which by stimulating adrenal steroid secretion, including corticosteroids and estrogens, enhances the effect of the ovarian hormones.

Adrenal Cortex

Cortisol is necessary for galactopoiesis. In addition, in at least some species, corticosteroids contribute to breast growth and development. Also, in some species complete bilateral adrenalectomy is necessary to induce complete breast atrophy, possibly due to withdrawal of estrogen as well as other steroids secreted by the adrenal cortex.

Testosterone

The role of androgens in breast growth and development appears to vary with the stage of development, age and the endocrine status. Its role in morphogenesis of the breast in the fetus has been mentioned above. During the reproductive years androgens, when present in larger than physiologic amounts, tend to inhibit mammary growth, development and lactation. This is generally assumed to be an antiestrogenic action. However, when estrogen levels are very low, some mammary proliferation may result, probably due to partial conversion of androgens to estrogens. The administration of androgens to the male, for example, may induce gynecomastia. It has also been claimed that androgen may potentiate the action of progesterone on the mammary acini.

Thyroid

Laboratory studies have shown that in some species thyroidectomized animals do not have as good breast development as controls. The administration of thyroid hormone to these animals, when all other factors are intact, results in improved breast development. The effect of thyroid hormone is generally believed to be due to potentiation of the effect of the ovarian steroids rather than a direct morphogenetic action.

Insulin

Insulin, which is known to be of importance in the process of lactogenesis, also serves a permissive role in maintaining the integrity of the ductal and alveolar systems. This is generally attributed to a favorable general influence of insulin on metabolic activity of mammary tissue rather than a direct or specific effect. This is supported by in vitro isotopic metabolic studies following the addition of insulin to incubation media containing mammary tissue slices.

Placental Hormones

The placenta, because of its secretion of large amounts of a number of hormones, plays a major role in inducing maximal alveolar development of the breasts and in preparing the breasts for lactation. Estrogen and progesterone rise progressively to reach very high titers at term. Human placental lactogen (human chorionic somatomammotropin), a protein hormone with both growth hormone and lactogenic hormone properties, increases in proportion to the weight of the placenta. During pregnancy there is also a moderate increase in the level of pituitary prolactin. Human chorionic gonadotropin, which rises dramatically during the early weeks of gestation, tends to increase breast development by its luteotropic action on the ovary; whether it also exerts a direct effect on the breast is not known. Relaxin has been found to have a stimulating effect on mammary development in laboratory rodents.

Hormonology of Lactation

Lactopoiesis and the maintenance of lactation are dependent on a number of hormones in addition to those required for the preparatory growth and development of the duct and acinar tissue. Of these, prolactin is the most important. However, in most species, the rabbit being a possible exception, prolactin alone will not initiate lactation, unless adrenocortical steroids are also present. Of these, the most important synergist in the human is cortisol, although in laboratory animals corticosterone

VANDERBILT MEDICAL CENTER LIBRARY

is almost as effective. Insulin and human placental lactogen also exert a positive influence in lactopoiesis. Oxytocin plays an important role as the milk let-down factor.

The hormonal changes that occur during pregnancy exert a particularly positive influence on the secretory activity of the breasts. There is a marked and progressive rise in estrogen and progesterone, both of which reach their peak values at term, stimulating maximal alveolar development of the breasts. During the early weeks of gestation the estrogen and progesterone come chiefly from the corpus luteum, which is maintained by the rising titers of human chorionic gonadotropin plus the additional luteotropic action of HPL. Subsequently, the placenta secretes these steroids. Human placental lactogen also rises progressively during gestation. This hormone, having both lactogenic and growth hormone activity, favors breast parenchymal growth. During pregnancy there is also an increased secretion of prolactin by the pituitary. However, despite the increase in prolactin and HPL, lactation does not occur during pregnancy. This is attributed to the high level of estrogen and to a lesser degree of progesterone, which are believed to inhibit the action of prolactin on the breasts. This is explained by the decrease in prolactin receptors which results from the high levels of estrogen and progesterone. Following delivery of the placenta, estrogen and progesterone levels drop abruptly so that the prolactin effect can predominate.

The action of prolactin is dependent on binding by prolactin receptors in the breast epethelial cells. This initiates the biochemical events leading to milk secretion.

Once initiated, nursing maintains lactation through the well-known neuroendocrine suckling reflex. Stimuli from the nipple are transmitted via mammary nerve tracts up the spinal cord, to the brain, then to the hypothalamus, with the subsequent release of hypothalamic neurohumors which favor lactation. One of the hypothalamic hormones stimulated by this afferent reflex arc is oxytocin, which acts upon the myoepithelial cells surrounding the mammary alveoli to force the milk into the duct system where it can be more easily obtained by suckling. Clinically, the secretion of oxytocin by this neuroendocrine reflex is also evidenced by the uterine contractions, or "after pains," that often occur during nursing.

Prolactin-Inhibiting Factors

The control of prolactin secretion by the pituitary is influenced through the hypothalamus by means of stimulating or inhibiting neurohumors. In the human, inhibition is the main factor and is mediated by prolactin-inhibiting factor (PIF). This thesis is supported by the fact that when the adenohypophysis is freed from hypothalamic influence by complete severance of the stalk, including the portal vascular cirulation, prolactin levels increase. FSH and LH, dependent upon hypothalamic GnRH, of course decrease following stalk section, a combination which readily explains the occurrence of amenorrhea and galactorrhea after stalk section by surgery or other lesions destroying the portal vascular connections.

PIF is believed to be a small polypeptide. Its exact nature is not yet known, but may be identical with dopamine or a substance released by dopamine, in that prolactin inhibition can be achieved by dopamine and dopaminergic drugs such as L-dopa. Certain ergot compounds, including bromocriptine, can inhibit lactation and lower prolactin levels. Bromocriptine (Parlodel) is now widely used clinically in hyperprolactinemia syndromes, and more recently has been approved for lactation inhibition in postpartum women.

Estrogen alone or in conjunction with progesterone, as in the oral contraceptives, or estrogen and androgen combinations have long been used to inhibit lactation in postpartum women. The mechanism here appears to be similar to that in pregnancy, namely to cause a decrease in prolactin receptors and thus interfere with the action of prolactin at a local level.

Norepinephrine and epinephrine are mild inhibitors of prolactin, as are the monoamine oxidase inhibitors, and some cholinergic drugs, such as acetylcholine.

Prolactin-Stimulating Factors

Although inhibition through a presumed PIF appears to be the chief element in the physiologic control of prolactin secretion by the pituitary hormones, stimulation of prolactin, at least under certain circumstances, has been documented. Whether an actual, specific hypothalamic prolactin-releasing factor (PRF) exists in the human is not known. However, it is to be noted that TRH, the thyroid-releasing hormone, which when administered increases TSH, also increases prolactin, and may thus act as a physiologic prolactin-stimulating hormone. On the other hand, the observation that, during periods of stress, prolactin levels may increase without an increase in TSH suggests that there may be two distinct factors.

Estrogen is also a known stimulator of prolactin. This may account for the observation that in occasional women glactorrhea may occur during the use of oral contraceptives. Ordinarily, however, there is enough estrogen in the oral contraceptives to interfere with the binding of prolactin and thus to inhibit milk secretion.

There are also pharmacologic stimulators of prolactin secretion which may result in galactorrhea. These include inhibitors of dopamine, such as alpha-methyldopa; inhibitors of dopamine action, such as the phenothiazines and reserpine compounds; certain biologic amines, such as serotonin; the pineal hormone, melatonin, and its precursor tryptophan. Recently it has been shown that the opioid peptides may also have this action of causing galactorrhea, with or without menstrual dysfunction, as noted in some marijuana users.

Physical stimulation of the afferent nerves from the breast to spinal cord, other than by normal nursing, may also stimulate prolactin secretion and lactation. Persistent sexual stimulation of the nipples is not an uncommon cause for a turbid or milky secretion, and is usually not accompanied by menstrual dysfunction. Suckling of a child by a nonpregnant woman may induce lactation and, indeed, in some instances adoptive mothers have successfully nursed. There are also rare reports of successful nursing of an infant by a male. Injuries to the chest wall which affect the mammary nerves may induce a milky discharge as has been reported after incisions, gall bladder operations, burns and herpes zoster. Emotional and other psychic factors also occasionally produce hyperprolactinemia and lactation. For example, it is known that a woman does not actually have to nurse her baby to have an elevation in her prolactin level. Even the sight of her baby or hearing the hungry baby may initiate the change. Stress, too, is believed in some instances to result in an amenorrhea-galactorrhea syndrome.

Bibliography

Botella-Llusia, J.: Endocrinology of Woman. Philadelphia, London, Toronto:W. B. Saunders Co., 1973, pp. 463-482.

Cowie, H.T. and Folley, S.J.: The mammary gland and lactation. *In* Young, W.C. (ed.): Sex and Internal Secretions, ed. 3. Baltimore: Williams & Wilkins Co., 1961, vol. 2, pp. 590-642.

Nagasawa, H. and Yanai, R.: Normal and abnormal growth of the mammary gland. *In* Yokoyama, A., Mizumo, H. and Nagasawa, H. (eds.): Physiology of Mammary Glands. Tokyo and Baltimore:Japan Scientific Societies Press and University Park Press, 1978.

Meites, J.: Neuroendocrinology of lactation. J. Invest. Dermatol. 63:119-124, 1974.

Reyniak, J.V.: Physiology of the breast. *In* Gallager, H.S., Leis, H.P., Jr., Snyderman, R.K. and Urban, J.A. (eds.): The Breast. St. Louis:C. V. Mosby Co., 1978, pp. 23-32.

Vorheer, H.: The Breast Morphology. Physiology and Lactation. New York, San Francisco, London:Academic Press, 1974.

Self-Evaluation Quiz

1. Progesterone is the hormone chiefly responsible for the development of the ductal system of the breast.
   a) True
   b) False

2. Prolactin-inhibiting factor is a pituitary hormone that inhibits lactation.
   a) True
   b) False

3. The breast epithelium undergoes cyclic changes during the menstrual cycle.
   a) True
   b) False

4. Stimulation of the nipple during breast feeding stimulates secretion of prolactin and oxytocin.
   a) True
   b) False

5. Human placental lactogen is a steroid hormone secreted by the placenta which stimulates breast growth.
   a) True
   b) False

6. In the human the hormone chiefly responsible for regulation of prolactin is:
   a) Progesterone
   b) Luteinizing hormone
   c) Prolactin-inhibiting factor
   d) Prolactin-releasing factor
   e) Chorionic somatomammotropin

7. Transection of the pituitary stalk produces an amenorrhea-
   galactorrhea syndrome by:
   a) Lowering PIF
   b) Lowering gonadotropins
   c) Raising thyrotropin-releasing hormone
   d) Lowering growth hormone
   e) Increasing prolactin-releasing hormone
8. Hormones which are known to stimulate growth and
   development of the breast include:
   a) Estrogen
   b) Progesterone
   c) Corticosteroids
   d) Prolactin
   e) Thyroxine
9. Hyperprolactinemia often occurs in which of the following
   conditions:
   a) Chiari-Frommel syndrome
   b) Simmond-Sheehan syndrome
   c) Pituitary microadenomas
   d) Cushing syndrome
   e) Anorexia nervosa
10. Drugs that inhibit prolactin include which of the following:
   a) Reserpine
   b) Chlorpromazine
   c) Bromocriptine
   d) L-dopa
   e) Thyroxine

Answers on page 335.

Pathology of Benign Breast Disease

Arthur S. Patchefsky, M.D.

Objective

The purpose of this paper is to discuss the component parts of cystic disease in relation to their importance as markers for subsequent development of carcinoma, with emphasis on the need for close liaison between the surgeon, mammographer and pathologist in the management of these patients.

It is important to separate fibrocystic disease into its component histological parts. In most institutions it has been used as a diagnostic wastebasket for almost any piece of benign breast tissue that the surgeon removes from the female breast, with the exception, of course, of more precisely defined lesions, such as fibroadenomas or papillomas. There is increasing evidence that not all of the component parts of fibrocystic disease are equally as important as histological markers to identify women with a propensity to develop breast cancer.

Anatomically, most of the spectrum of lesions that we recognize as fibrocystic disease actually occurs at the terminal portion of the breast lobule. Both the epithelial components of fibrocystic disease (florid adenosis, papillomatosis, blunt duct adenosis) and the nonproliferative types of fibrocystic disease, the cysts themselves, arise in the terminal lobe and terminal lobular duct. The solitary intraductal papilloma, the subareolar papilloma, and some intraductal papillomatosis take origin from the larger and intermediate-diameter collecting ducts.

The lobule consists of multiple separate acini or glands which make up the secretory portion of the breast, as well as

Arthur S. Pathchefsky, M.D., Professor of Pathology, Jefferson Medical College; Director, Surgical Pathology, Thomas Jefferson University Hospital, Philadelphia, Pa.

the terminal collecting ductule and its associated stroma which separates it from the intralobular stroma, or the stroma between the lobules of the breast.

The acini contain a single layer of regular cells surrounded by a layer of flattened cells which abut on the basement membrane. These have been shown by ultrastructual and immunological techniques to be myoepithelial cells, or cells which combine the structure and functional features of both smooth muscle cells and epithelial cells. These cells are probably important in the histogenesis of certain components of cystic disease, particularly sclerosing adenosis.

One of the most common types of nonproliferative fibrocystic disease that we pathologists see is what we call in my institution fibrous mastopathy. This is a condition in which the epithelial lobule and terminal duct system becomes transformed into a firm mass of rather dense connective tissue. The epithelium becomes atrophic and eventually is squeezed out and disappears, with the exception of a few residual epithelial and/or myoepithelial cells. This is most commonly a condition of older women. It represents an involutional process within the breast. We occasionally see it to a lesser degree in younger women when it causes a palpable mass in the breast. This lesion has not been associated statistically with an increased risk for breast cancer.

In the classical form of fibrocystic disease, we see macrocysts or gross cysts, the typical blue dome cysts of Bloodgood. These are the types of cysts which are frequently aspirated by the surgeon rather than biopsied.

Apocrine metaplasia is histologically similar to the apocrine sweat glands and ultrastructually it is very much analogous to that type of epithelium. Not only cysts but all types of benign lesions and sometimes malignant breast tumors may show this change.

Sclerosing adenosis is a very common component of the fibrocystic disease picture. In fact, I would say that the majority of patients who have biopsies for what is purported to be fibrocystic disease, along with cysts, have a focal area of sclerosing adenosis microscopically present. However, to the surgeon and to the mammographer, the term usually means a mass lesion which is produced by a localized proliferation of sclerosing adenosis.

This is commonly seen in younger women. Indeed, there are some young women whose breasts become filled with this proliferating adenosis. Haagensen has referred to this as adenosis tumor. We call these cases florid adenosis, or the florid phase of sclerosing adenosis. These young women usually have lumpy breasts, they are frequently biopsied, and the propensity of sclerosing adenosis to calcify makes it very common for these women to have frequent mammograms. However, as with fibrous mastopathy and certain of the other types of benign proliferations, this lesion has not been associated with any increased risk of carcinoma, but, rather, there is a very real risk — mammographically, clinically and pathologically — of mistaking this lesion for carcinoma of the breast.

As the lesion matures, and the condition presists, there is a tendency for the stromal portion or the connective tissue to become more prominent and the glands to decrease in number. As the connective tissue increases and the glands decrease, the lesion can be transformed into a hard mass which can mimic an infiltrating carcinoma.

Duct papillomatosis is another proliferative lesion of the mammary parenchyma, usually a very common component of fibrocystic disease. Occasionally, it is seen by itself without other components of fibrocystic disease. It consists of an irregular proliferation of ductal epithelium in the small and medium-sized ductules of the breast. Generally, this is over a wide field in the breast, but occasionally it is localized. It is a disease of women aged 35 to 55 years. Sometimes, it can be difficult to differentiate microscopically from carcinoma.

Diffuse intraductal papillomatosis should be differentiated from large-duct papilloma. This is a large, grossly visible tumor which arises usually in the subareolar area or in the collecting ducts rather than in the medium-sized or terminal ducts. It is grossly visible and is often clinically palpable, giving rise to nipple discharge.

There is some controversy about this in the literature, but a solitary papilloma of the breast probably does not indicate a woman who is at increased risk for breast cancer. However, this is probably not the case for women who have multiple intraductal papillomas of the breast, particularly those in which the papillomas are bilateral.

A variant of intraductal papilloma is the subareolar papilloma. Frequently, these lesions have a rather florid sclerosing reaction to the papillary proliferation. Again, this is one of the types of lesions which may be misdiagnosed pathologically and at times clinically as carcinoma of the breast, particularly since not only nipple discharge but itching eczematous reactions of the nipple may sometimes be seen which may mimic the clinical features of Paget disease.

Duct ectasia is an inflammatory reaction in which there is an initial periductal inflammatory reaction which then causes secondary changes within the larger ducts, which eventually become fibrotic, distended and filled with cellular debris. This is commonly associated with nipple discharge. This is not associated with an increased risk for carcinoma.

Whenever we are faced with a frozen section or biopsy of a breast, we tell our residents to ask themselves, when they are considering the diagnosis of malignancy, can this lesion be papilloma, papillomatosis, florid adenosis or some other type of benign proliferation? In a review of cases screened at our institution in the mammography screening center, out of 407 biopsies there were only two which were overdiagnosed as malignancy. These were by pathologists who had seen the material before we reviewed it. Both of those lesions showed florid adenosis. One was a case of florid adenosis with an associated lobular carcinoma in situ, so that was not a complete miss, but this patient had a radical mastectomy. The other was an example of florid and sclerosing adenosis without cancer, for which the patient had radical mastectomy. So some of these lesions can be rather confusing and warrant careful microscopic study.

Atypical lobular hyperplasia is a lesion which involves the terminal lobule and the terminal duct. Qualitatively, individual cells match up fairly well with the individual cells of lobular carcinoma in situ. This process, however, lacks the same monotony and uniformity and the ability to distend the terminal ducts and lobules by a proliferation of these cells.

However, even though this lesion is somewhat less than what we can confidently regard morphologically as lobular carcinoma in situ, there is increasing evidence that it is probably an incompletely developed form of lobular carcinoma in situ, based upon, first, the frequent association of this lesion with fully developed lobular carcinoma and, second, the fact that in follow-up studies of patients with only this lesion a significant increase has been shown in the incidence of carcinoma of the breast, which is only slightly less than that of the fully developed lobular carcinoma in situ.

Similarly, in atypical ductal hyperplasia, the medium-sized ducts participate in an epithelial proliferative process which has some but not all of the histologic features of intraductal carcinoma of the breast.

We have shown some evidence that these atypical lesions are associated with breast cancer. In asymptomatic women who were referred for mammographic screening, 8% (31 out of 258) of otherwise benign biopsies showed either atypical lobular hyperplasia or atypical papillomatosis of the breast. When we compared that to 51 mastectomy specimens which were examined in our own laboratory from the same group of women who had cancer of the breast, 28% (14 of 51) of these women had similar atypias of the breast. This is a highly significant incidence of atypical proliferative disease of the breast associated with breast cancer in this group of women. Interestingly, there appeared to be no correlation between the other types of benign cystic disease and breast cancer in our mastectomies.

In summary, clinicians, pathologists and breast surgeons should think in terms of separating the component parts of cystic disease into their proliferative and nonproliferative components, and particularly into subsets that have increasingly been shown to be important as markers for the subsequent development of carcinoma. For this reason, a close liaison between the surgeon, mammographer and the pathologist should be developed for meaningful correlations and for intelligent follow-up of these patients.

Bibliography

Page, D.L., Vander Zwagg, R., Rogers, L.W. et al: Relation between component parts of fibrocystic disease complex and breast cancer. JNCI 61:1055-1063, 1978.

Patchefsky, A.S., Shaber, G.S., Schwartz, G.F. et al: The pathology of breast cancer detected by mass population screening. Cancer 40:1659-1670, 1977.

Self-Evaluation Quiz

1. All components of fibrocystic disease are equally important in identifying women at risk for breast cancer.
   a) True
   b) False
2. Most fibrocystic disease originates in the terminal lobule.
   a) True
   b) False
3. Fibrous mastopathy has not been associated with increased cancer risk.
   a) True
   b) False
4. Which of the following may show apocrine metaplasia?
   a) Cysts
   b) Various benign lesions
   c) Malignant breast tumors
   d) All of the above
5. Infiltrating carcinoma is often mimicked by:
   a) Intraductal papillomatosis
   b) Sclerosing adenosis
   c) Apocrine metaplasia
6. Nipple discharge and itching eczematous reactions are typical of:
   a) Duct ectasia
   b) Florid adenosis
   c) Subareolar papilloma
7. Evidence suggests that atypical lobular hyperplasia is an incompletely developed form of lobular carcinoma in situ.
   a) True
   b) False

Answers on page 335.

Methylxanthines in Breast Disease

John P. Minton, M.D., Ph.D.

Objective

The most common disease of the female breast is described clinically as fibrocystic disease. An effective treatment of this disease for many patients consuming methylxanthines and nicotine is total and complete abstention from methylxanthine consumption and nicotine use. The effect of stopping, cutting down and continuing methylxanthine and nicotine consumption will be presented. Methylxanthines are found in coffee, tea, colas, chocolate and many prescription and nonprescription medications.

In 1972, I was asked to speak before the American Cancer Society's meeting for science writers. My topic at that time was to present the initial work I had done with L-dopa as a suppressor of serum prolactin in patients with metastatic breast cancer which was producing serious bone pain. I reported that the use of L-dopa induced bone pain relief as an indicator for endocrine manipulative surgery. At that same meeting, the concept of studying cyclic adenosine monophosphate (cAMP) in breast cancer tissue was proposed by Dr. E. W. Sutherland, who had recently received the Nobel Prize for his work with cAMP, the second messenger in cellular information. This background really puts things into perspective as to the time and the work that has been done in developing the data to be reported in this presentation.

John P. Minton, M.D., Ph.D., Professor of Surgery and American Cancer Society Professor of Clinical Oncology, Department of Surgery, The Ohio State University College of Medicine, Columbus.

This study is supported by The Ohio State University Development Fund 532809, the Grand Chapter of Ohio Order of the Eastern Star and Phi Beta Psi Sorority.

We soon began measuring cAMP in human breast cancer. Over the next few years considerable data were gathered. After an initial analysis, cAMP was found to be high when compared to the levels in fibrocystic disease tissue, and very high when compared to normal tissue levels. Biopsied tissue specimens were immediately placed in liquid nitrogen, and then cAMP and cGMP determinations were made. A comparison between the cancer tissue, normal tissue and benign fibrocystic disease tissue began to show a difference in the cAMP and cGMP average values for the different kinds of breast disease entities, with significant differences between the levels in normal tissue, benign breast disease and breast cancer. The next question that needed to be answered was, what makes cAMP go up in diseased breast tissue cells? In normal breast tissue cells the values were low, in fibrocystic disease the values were moderately elevated, and in cancer cells they were markedly elevated.

There are many factors that influence cAMP levels. One way to increase cAMP is to block its breakdown mechanism. A major breakdown mechanism is by the phosphodiesterase enzyme which changes cAMP to the inactive form, 5'-AMP, in a fraction of a second. A well-known class of agents which block the breakdown of cAMP through their action as phosphodiesterase inhibitors is the methylxanthines. Methylxanthines include caffeine, theophylline and theobromine. *Caffeine* is found in coffee. Depending upon how the coffee is brewed, the concentration of caffeine varies considerably. Most Americans consume between 50 and 100 mg of caffeine in each cup of coffee. Made Brazilian style, coffee may contain up to 300 mg of caffeine per demitasse. The cola drinks available today generally have about 50 to 70 mg per 12-ounce can or bottle. There are also a number of soft drinks which are not called colas but which have caffeine in them. Tea usually contains both *theophylline* and *caffeine*. It will vary depending upon how long one steeps or brews the leaves. Chocolate contains *theobromine* and *caffeine*. Theobromine has been a particularly difficult biochemical agent to measure and only recently have we been able to do that accurately. Clearly, chocolate chip cookies, hot chocolate, candy bars, chocolate milk, etc. contain some complement of theobromine and caffeine. Asthmatic medicines contain theophylline. Caffeine is a component of a number of pain medications. Weekend headaches may be due to caffeine deficiency in people who have a physiologic dependence on this chemical.

The biochemistry is relatively simple. ATP is the high-energy source. The enzyme adenylate cyclase changes the ATP to cAMP. This is normally available as a transient second messenger. Certain cyclic AMP molecules in the breast's physiologic chemistry then stimulate a second molecule known as a protein kinase. These protein kinases may have two molecular directions: one would direct breast epithelial cells to make fluid, and another protein kinase molecule may direct breast tissue cells to proliferate fibroblasts, thereby increasing fibrous tissue. Depending upon the age of the patient, different types of pathology are found. Younger women (postpubertal) tend to make dense fibrous tissue. Women in their late 20s or 30s and early 40s tend to make some combination of cystic fluid and fibrous tissue. This response may occur even into the mid-60s in some women. The breakdown of cAMP by phosphodiesterase is an instantaneous type of reaction, and cAMP is transformed to the inactive form, $5'$-AMP. If the phosphodiesterase enzyme breakdown of cAMP is obstructed through the inhibitory effect of methylxanthines, then the transfer of cAMP from the secondary messenger state to the inactive form of $5'$-AMP does not occur. As a result, the breast tissue cells continue to receive instruction from the protein kinases, and the breast cells dutifully continue to make fluid and fibrous tissues, leading to the development of a pathologic entity generally called fibrocystic disease of the breast.

Now, the first part of this cAMP equation also becomes the second part of the pathologic problem. Biochemical factors that influence the activation of adenylate cyclase and hence cAMP production include hormones and catecholamines and biacetyls. Therefore, the levels of sex hormones released into the circulation in a cyclic pattern with the menstrual cycle also influence the amount of cAMP being made at any given time. Women may develop some tenderness and swelling of breast tissue as hormone elevations stimulate cAMP and protein kinase release. An additional clinical problem with the adenylate cyclase portion of the equation is that women who use tobacco absorb enough nicotine to biochemically activate a release of norepinephrine and epinephrine; this in turn releases adenylate cyclase, which makes additional cAMP and thereby stimulates the protein kinases to direct the breast tissue to respond. The combination of nicotine stimulation and inhibition of the cAMP breakdown system by methylxanthines magnifies the problem.

Our original data were reported to the Society of University Surgeons in 1979 [1]. In the initial observations, 47 patients who had segmental or diffuse, unilateral or bilateral fibrocystic breast disease did not have cyclic or intermittent breast involvement. Their disease had been present for some time and persisted between menstrual periods. Some women were considering subcutaneous mastectomies for the relief of pain. Many women could not sleep on their abdomen because of breast pain. When a careful evaluation of the methylxanthine consumption of these women was obtained and evaluated, an average of 190 mg of caffeine was found to be consumed per day. Some individuals were consuming more than a gram per 24 hours. Mammograms, echograms and needle biopsies were obtained to confirm that there was no malignancy, in addition to a careful physical examination performed by two or more examiners. Many of these women had previous breast biopsies.

Patients who have been followed clinically report that pain relief usually occurred first, sometimes as soon as one week after *total cessation* of caffeine consumption. The earliest changes occurred in younger women. Many women 40 years of age and older required 12 months for a clinically detectable change. If women did not totally abstain from consuming methylxanthines, resolution of the disease was slow and patients became discouraged. Absolute and total abstention from the consumption of methylxanthine-containing agents must occur for a satisfactory clinical response. Mammography was very slow to change. In most patients demonstrable changes occurred only after 12 months of total abstention. Echograms were difficult to interpret but occasionally were very effective in documenting measurable changes in breast pathology. Of the 47 women studied, 20 stopped methylxanthine consumption. Thirteen of these 20 had complete resolution of their disease. Twenty-seven of the 47 women could not stop methylxanthine consumption and only one improved significantly.

One benefit that happens when a patient abstains from methylxanthine consumption and her clinical disease resolves is that a biopsy is not necessary to confirm malignancy in the breast. Her lesions are gone and the symptomatology which led her to seek help is gone. On the other hand, if the clinical disease is persistent after eight weeks' observation, a biopsy is performed to confirm that the disease is only fibrocystic disease.

Since the original report, more patient data have been obtained. There are now 45 women who have stopped methylxanthine consumption. Of these 45 women, 37 have had complete resolution of their disease, 7 have shown improvement and 1 patient has remained unchanged. Of 28 patients who decreased their methylxanthine consumption, 7 experienced resolution of their disease, 14 were clinically improved and 7 were unchanged. When patients continued the same amount of methylxanthine consumption, only 2 of 12 had resolution of their disease, 1 patient improved and 9 remained unimproved. The increased number of clinical observations continues to directly correlate methylxanthine consumption and fibrocystic disease. When patients were both methylxanthine and nicotine consumers, and they stopped consumption of both agents, 16 of 20 patients had complete resolution of their disease and the other 4 were clinically improved; none remained unchanged. When women stopped only their methylxanthine consumption but continued to smoke cigarettes, 5 of 7 improved and 2 were unchanged. When they decreased both methylxanthine and nicotine consumption, 1 of 3 improved but 2 showed no improvement. When patients continued both at the same amount, 3 of 3 showed no improvement.

In women whose breast disease had not resolved completely or had not made a significant clinical improvement by the eight-week check-up, a biopsy was carried out.

It is important to stress that any patient who stops methylxanthine consumption as a method to treat her breast disease must first have a physician's opinion that the disease is benign, and, secondly, the course of the disease must be followed by a responsible physician so that a malignancy is not overlooked.

Forty-eight patients who stopped methylxanthine consumption, but had not significantly improved in eight weeks, had a confirmatory biopsy of their benign breast disease. Thirty-eight of these 48 women now have had complete resolution of the clinical disease in their breasts. Ten have improved clinically and none remain unchanged. Nineteen patients continued both methylxanthine and nicotine consumption after they had had a confirmatory benign biopsy, and all remained unchanged.

Conclusion

A group of 106 women with fibrocystic breast disease were requested to abstain totally from methylxanthine consumption and nicotine use. In 68% of these women disease was resolved. In an additional 24% the clinical disease improved when they decreased their consumption of methylxanthines and use of nicotine. Eighty-four percent of the patients observed who could not stop or cut down on methylxanthine consumption had unimproved breast disease. One hundred percent of those who could not stop or cut down their smoking and methylxanthine consumption had unimproved breast disease.

Reference

1. Minton, J.P., Foecking, M.K., Webster, D.J.T. and Matthews, R.H.: Caffeine, cyclic nucleotides, and breast disease. Surgery 86:105-109, 1979.

Self-Evaluation Quiz

1. The breakdown of cAMP is interfered with by methylxanthines.
   a) True
   b) False
2. Methylxanthines are readily available in dietary products.
   a) True
   b) False
3. Two thirds of patients with benign fibrocystic disease will have resolution of their clinical disease by total and permanent abstention from methylxanthine consumption.
   a) True
   b) False
4. Nicotine consumption increases the production of cAMP.
   a) True
   b) False

5. Some breast lumps which appear to be benign fibrocystic disease may be cancer.
   a) True
   b) False
6. An evaluation of a breast with suspected fibrocystic disease may require needle aspiration, mammography or open biopsy to rule out cancer.
   a) True
   b) False

Answers on page 335.

Breast Cancer — Treatment and Pretreatment Considerations

Breast Cancer Screening — Thermography's Role

Gary S. Shaber, M.D.

Objective

This paper presents a comparison of mammography, clinical examination and thermography to assess their effectiveness as an initial screening method.

Introduction

In June 1973 a cooperative research program was begun under National Cancer Institute funding by Thomas Jefferson University and the Health Insurance Plan of Greater New York to determine whether thermography might play a role in the early detection of breast cancer through screening of large population groups. Implementation of this cooperative project was the result of an earlier program conducted by the Health Insurance Plan of Greater New York evaluating the role of x-ray mammography in the early detection of breast cancer in asymptomatic women.

Although the two projects had the same objectives and basic methods of procedure, there were certain significant differences. Primarily, the Health Insurance Plan of Greater New York's program would examine 20,000 women previously enrolled in the insurance plan and the Jefferson program would solicit 20,000 asymptomatic volunteers from the general population of the Philadelphia metropolitan area. In addition, the Health Insurance Plan program would examine and follow up all patients at hospitals cooperating in their program and the Jefferson volunteers could be followed at any institution within the metropolitan area, whether affiliated or unaffiliated with Thomas Jefferson University.

Gary S. Shaber, M.D., Research Professor of Radiology, Breast Diagnostic Center, Thomas Jefferson University, Philadelphia, Pa.

Background

Approximately 35,000 new cases of breast cancer will be discovered in the United States this year. These cancers will occur for the most part in the 40 million women in the risk age group (40 to 75). Nearly 90% of these cancers will be found by the woman herself, and over 60% of them will be noticed at an advanced stage [1]. In spite of increased use of self-examination and advances in techniques such as mammography and thermography, there has been essentially no reduction in the death rate from breast cancer for the past 50 years [2]. Until a preventive program is developed, the greatest hope for reduction of breast cancer mortality lies in early discovery by mass screening of the adult at-risk female population. Experience has shown that improved ten-year survival can be obtained when the disease is discovered early and is still localized to the breast [3]. Several methods of early detection have been investigated by the National Cancer Institute. They involve screening of large numbers of women with different physical diagnostic modalities in the hope of identifying high-risk groups and/or patients currently with the disease at an early stage.

Of all the screening tests that have been employed: x-ray mammography, physical examination and thermography, x-ray mammography appears to be the most efficacious in the discovery of early carcinomas of the breast. Approximately 90% of extant breast cancer, with 50% of these confined to the breast, can be discovered by x-ray mammography screening [4]. However, evidence exists suggesting that the increased radiation burden to the population, when large numbers of women are screened with x-ray mammography, may be harmful [5]. This potential risk of repetitive screening of the adult female population has prompted a search for alternative noninvasive physical techniques which could substitute for x-ray mammography. Thermography was seen as one potential candidate.

The physical principles of thermography have been studied by many investigators [6-8]. The amount of infrared energy emitted from the body depends on the absolute temperature of the skin surface and its emissivity [9], and is described by Planck's radiation law. Measurements by Hardy [10] and by Watmough and Oliver [11] have shown that the emissivity of skin lies between 0.98 and 1.00, and therefore human skin is a nearly perfect absorber and emitter of infrared energy. The majority of medical thermographic scanners are sensitive only to radiation in the 2- to 14μ wavelength range [10]. Dreyfus [12] derived the equation describing the amount of energy detected by a thermography over narrow emission bands.

The thermal patterns of the female breast have been studied by many investigators. Fay and Henny [13], and later Lawson [14], reported that the skin surface over malignant tumors in the breast was usually between 1° and 3°C warmer than the surrounding skin. No corresponding temperature elevation was detectable over benign tumors. These findings were confirmed by Lloyd-Williams et al and others [15, 16]. The cause of the temperature increase is still not fully understood. Carcinomas of the breast are metabolically active, and the veins that drain these tumors are generally hotter than normal [17] and could account for at least part of the temperature elevation at the skin surface. Lawson and Gaston [17] demonstrated that the temperature of mammary tumors exceeds that of the local arterial and venous blood. The venous blood is warmer than the arterial, indicating that the latter serves as a coolant and that the transfer of heat to the other parts of the breast occurs as a process of venous convection. Since the superficial and deep venous systems of the breast unite in the plexus of Haller immediately behind the areola, it is possible that blood draining from a tumor may be shunted to any part of the breast. For this reason a positive breast thermogram may consist of exaggeration of all or part of the superficial venous system or isolated warming of the areola. Since the surface manifestations of the heat exchange are dependent upon the tissue depth of the veins as well as the temperature of the blood circulating within them, the disparities between location of the abnormal signal and the tumor are readily understandable [18].

In the screening of symptomatic women, most investigators have found this tool to be very useful. However, in many of the studies thermography was not performed independent of other examinations and controlled verification of thermography's findings was not included. Several of these studies are summarized in Table 1.

Because of the encouraging anecdotal findings by previous investigators of thermography's ability to detect breast cancer, an objective screening program was established utilizing x-ray mammography, physical examination and thermography to test

Table 1. Summary of Screening Studies of Symptomatic Women

Investigator	No. of Patients	No. of Tumors	Thermography False-Positive Rate	Thermography True-Positive Rate
Davey et al [19]	1,717	15	11.5%	73%
Isard et al [20]	2,696	55	31%	72%
Stark & Way [21]	5,234	27	–	71%
Dowdy [22]	1,950	57	17%	73%
Tricoire [23]	300	78	5%	93%
Dodd [24]	4,726	197	11%	85%
Isard [25]	10,000	306	–	71%
Furnival [26]	414	77	15%	50%

this hypothesis. In this study 17,543 women between the ages of 45 and 65 were examined over a five-year period, using a combination of thermography, mammography and physical examination. The entire screening procedure took approximately 45 minutes and a detailed history was obtained prior to examination. The screening center could examine 60 patients per day. The objectives of the program were:

1. To determine whether thermography and clinical examination could be utilized as an initial screening procedure in lieu of mammography and clinical examination with no significant (10%) decrease in female breast cancer detection.

2. To determine whether the addition of thermography to an examination consisting of mammography and clinical examination would increase the detection rate by a significant amount (20%).

3. To determine whether thermography could be utilized to identify women with high risk of developing clinically demonstrable cancer of the breast within a time period of up to four years.

All examinations, with the exception of the physical examination, were interpreted independently by two readers and in cases of disagreement a third reading was performed and a conference held to resolve differences. The conference decision was not included in the statistical interpretation of the results of each examination. The physical examination was performed by a physician or trained nurse practitioner and any question-able finding was referred to the Director of Clinical Services for reexamination. The findings for every examination were computer encoded and the computer generated the final recommendations for each patient. Figure 1 shows the possible sequence of events, depending upon the results of the patient's initial examination.

Results

Number of Patients Examined

During the project period 17,543 patients were enrolled in the program and examined at least once with all modalities. There was a disproportionate number of white women in the

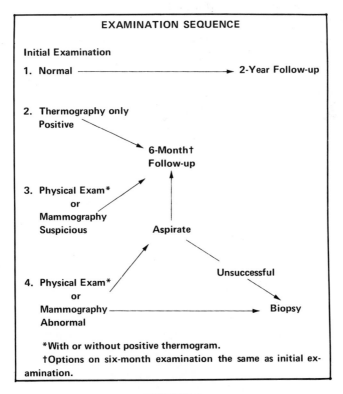

FIGURE 1.

program, relative to a random sampling of the population of women, aged 45 to 64, in the Philadelphia metropolitan area. However, there did not appear to be any significant bias toward a high-risk breast cancer age or religious group.

Total Number of Patient Visits

A total of 35,367 examinations using all modalities was performed on the 17,543 patients enrolled in the program, an average of about 2 examinations per patient. These examinations were performed during the three possible examination visits — initial, early recall (six-month follow-up) and biennial (two-year follow-up).

Response Rate to Breast Center Recommendations

Six-Month Follow-up Examinations (Early Recall). Some 10,934 six-month follow-up examinations were performed on 4,714 patients. The modality responsible for the six-month follow-up examination is given in Table 2. The preponderance

Table 2. Early Recall (Six-Months)
Recommendations by Modality on Initial Visit*

Positive Modality	No. of Patients	% of Patient Population
T only	2,911†	16.5
M only	865	4.9
C only	561	3.2
T–M	284	1.6
T–C	108	0.6
M–C	139	0.8
T–M–C	37	0.2
Total T	3,340	19.0
Total M	1,325	7.6
Total C	845	4.8
Total patients	4,714	26.9

T – Thermography.   M – Mammography.   C – Clinical examination.
*Total of 17,488 complete data files, 55 incomplete files (0.3%).
†Includes patients with thermography positive and other modality recommending biopsy.

of these requests was based on a positive thermographic examination alone. The total number of patients with an initial positive thermogram was 3,340, for a total thermographic positivity rate of 19%. Fifteen of these patients with a positive thermogram have subsequently been found to have an occult neoplasm, discovered during one of the six-month follow-up examinations. Seven hundred twenty-five patients did not return for six-month follow-up, comprising 15% of the six-month follow-up group and less than 4.5% of the total patient population. The majority of the patients, 438, who did not return for early recall examination were patients who were requested to return on the basis of positive thermography only.

Of the initial screened population, 1,325 (7.6%) were requested to return in six months as a result of a suspicious mammogram, and 845 patients (4.8%) were requested to return in six months because of a suspicious clinical examination.

Two-Year Follow-up Examinations. Of the 12,099 patients requested to have biennial examination, 6,890 (57%) returned. Table 3 details the response rate after the initial visit in the various follow-up categories.

Biopsy Recommendations

A total of 1,218 patients enrolled in the program had positive findings during the course of their protocol-dictated examinations. These findings, which required further follow-up, are summarized in Table 4.

A group of 322 patients had successful needle aspirations of cysts and required no further action other than the six-month follow-up. Of the 896 biopsies that were requested, 664

Table 3. Response Rate to Early Recall, Biennial Examination and Biopsy or Aspiration Request After Initial Screen

Recommendation	No. Requested	No. Returning	%
Early recall (6-month)	4,714	3,989*	85
Biennial examination	12,099	6,890	57
Biopsy or aspiration	693	574	83
Total	17,506†	11,453	65

*Number represents patients returning for first recall exam.
†Total of 37 incomplete data files (0.2%).

Table 4. Results of BDC Biopsy or Aspiration Request

Result	Visit Initial	Early Recall	Biennial	Total
Benign biopsy	266	166	24	456
Positive biopsy	152	31	25	208
Successful aspiration	144	165	13	322
Deferral	119	52	6	177
Incomplete case	12	6	37	55
Total	693	420	105	1,218

biopsies have been confirmed as being performed. For 55 (6.1%) of the 896 requested biopsies, data are incomplete and further follow-up is continuing. For various reasons, 177 requested biopsies were not performed. It was expected initially that the majority of the unperformed biopsies would be for patients who had clinically occult masses with a positive mammogram, or mammogram and thermogram. However, this was not the case, and the indications for the requested biopsies in both the performed and unperformed categories were similar. The reason for nonperformance of biopsy now appears to be primarily due to referring physician indifference to the recommendations of the Breast Diagnostic Center.

Tumors Discovered (10.4/1000)

One hundred eighty-three malignant breast lesions were discovered in the 615 patients who had biopsies performed after their initial or early recall visit, a quite favorable 30% positive biopsy to biopsy rate. Of these cancer cases 152 (83%) were discovered at initial screen and the remaining 31 (17%) were discovered on early recall (six-month visit). Table 5 reveals the distribution of these 183 tumors by age and prevalence and shows that our tumor patient population is not significantly biased by a high-incidence age group. This table also reveals that the number of tumors discovered (prevalence) in our population was significantly elevated above that which was projected, based upon the previous reported incidence rate for breast carcinoma in the United States population. Although our patient population was supposedly asymptomatic, the element of self-

Table 5. Distribution of Total Patient Population
and Tumors Discovered on Initial Visit and Early Recall

| | Tumors* (per 1000) | | Total Population‡ | |
Age	Discovered (Prevalence)	Incidence†	Actual	Expected§
45-49	7.3	1.56	5,042 (28.8%)	4,859 (27.7%)
50-54	9.0	1.68	5,135 (29.3%)	4,737 (27.0%)
55-59	12.0	1.88	4,180 (23.8%)	4,210 (24.0%)
60-64	17.9	2.22	2,790 (15.9%)	3,737 (21.3%)
Total	10.4	1.74‖	17,543	17,543

*Uncorrected for race and religion.
†Source: Third National Cancer Survey, NCI Monograph, 1975.
‡Total of 396 incomplete data files (2.2%).
§Source: U.S. Census, Philadelphia Metropolitan Area, 1970.
‖Corrected for actual population age distribution.

selection, also seen in other screening studies, cannot be ignored. The extent to which this factor biased the population was investigated through a questionnaire sent to the patients with proven tumors. Ninety-five percent of these patients responded and a surprisingly small percentage suspected that they had a breast lesion or ultimately were referred to our center because their physician suspected a tumor. The exclusion of these patients from the study would lower the tumor discovery rate in our population, but it would still remain three times the incidence rate. This high discovery rate is due to detection of prevalent tumors in the population prior to their time of natural manifestation, and as a result less than 25% of the tumor patients had nodal metastases at the time of biopsy, a rate one-half that normally expected.

Incident Cancers

Sixty-four proven carcinomas of the breast were discovered in our patient population following a negative initial screening examination. Twenty-eight of these cancers were detected at outside institutions (three patients had positive thermograms), 11 tumors were discovered at the Breast Diagnostic Center in patients who returned early without a scheduled examination because of the onset of symptoms, and an additional 25 of these cancers were discovered on a biennial screening examination (3.6/1000). The rate of 3.6 per thousand after a two-year interval approaches the normal incidence rate for a population of this age group. This incidence rate suggests that the initial screening examination was efficacious in removing most of the prevalent tumors from the population, with the possible exception of the additional 39 interval tumors discovered at outside institutions or at the Breast Diagnostic Center at unscheduled reexamination times. Retrospective examination of the x-ray mammograms on all interval carcinoma cases suggests that approximately 24% of these tumors could possibly have been detected at the time of initial examination.

The mean interval time between a negative examination and tumor discovery in these patients was 12.1 months. Only one of the interval cancers discovered at the Breast Diagnostic Center, either at biennial examination or in patients returning early because of symptoms, had significant lymph node metastasis (less than four nodes). The 12.1-month interval time between examination and discovery of the tumor would seem to imply that the two-year interval between screening examinations is too long for detection of small incident carcinomas. Table 6 summarizes the incidence of these interval carcinomas.

*Comparison of Modality Diagnostic
Accuracy*

Effectiveness of Each Modality in Breast Cancer Detection.
Table 7 reveals that since the start of our project, excluding

Table 6. Interval Cancers

Type	Number
Discovered on two-year follow-up	25
Discovered before two-year follow-up*	
(a) At Outside Institutions†	28
(b) At BDC‡	11
Total	64

*Mean interval time 12.1 ± 6.6 months.
†Three patients with BDC positive thermograms.
‡Patient returned early because of symptoms and previous exam was negative.

Table 7. Tumor Diagnosis at Breast Diagnostic Center
by Type of Examination – All Visits
(17,543 Patients)

| Modality | Tumors | | Total Positivity* | |
	No.	%	No.	%
Mammography	163 (154)†	78.3 (74.0)	1,880	10.7
Clincal	105 (98)†	50.5 (47.1)	1,293	7.4
Thermography	85 (90)†	40.9 (43.3)	3,603	20.5
Total	208	100.0	5,874	33.5

*Biopsy or early recall recommendation.
†Fifteen tumors only initially positive by thermography (7.2%).

non-two-year-follow-up interval cancers, x-ray mammography identified at time of biopsy 78.3% of the tumors, the highest percentage of all three examining modalities. Thermography was least sensitive, identifying 40.9% of the tumors. Clinical examination was able to identify only 50.5% of the lesions; thus, over 49% of the tumors were clinically occult small neoplasms with their associated favorable prognosis. Table 8 details the relative effectiveness of each modality for tumor discovery at the three different examination intervals: initial, early recall (six-month follow-up) and biennial (two-year follow-up). It can be seen that the effectiveness for both mammography and clinical examination in identifying tumors de-

Table 8. Modality Tumor Detection Rates (Percent)
at Each Examination Interval
(208 Tumors)

| Modality | Examination Interval | | | | |
	Initial	Recall	Initial & Recall	2-Year	All Visits
Mammography	79.6	64.5	77.1	88	78.3
Clinical	53.3	48.4	52.5	36	50.5
Thermography	42.1	54.8	44.3	16	40.9
T or C	69.7	78.1	71.6	48	68.8
T or M	86.8	77.4	85.3	88	85.6
M or C	100.0	100.0	100.0	100.0	100.0*

*Thirty-nine interval cancers with no biopsy recommendation are not included.

creases on the early recall examination, the effectiveness of mammography rises on the two-year follow-up, and that of clinical examination continues to fall. It is at this time that mammography's sensitivity is highest (88%). This is not the case for thermography, which shows a significant effectiveness in identifying tumors on early recall (54.8%) but is unable to show a significant sensitivity on two-year follow-up (16%). These results are probably explained by the inability of thermography and clinical examination to identify small early tumors.

Effectiveness of Thermography to Identify High-Risk Population. Fifteen patients would not have been recommended for biopsy (7.2% of the tumor cases) had not a positive thermogram required the patient to return in six months for further follow-up. In addition to the 15 cancer cases discovered at the Breast Diagnostic Center as a result of a positive thermogram, three Breast Diagnostic Center patients with positive thermograms had tumors discovered at outside institutions without Breast Diagnostic Center recommendations for biopsy. When the total thermographic positivity is considered, analysis of the number of additional tumors discovered by thermography fails to establish a significant difference from chance alone ($\chi^2 > 0.2$).

Since thermography alone recommended that 3,255 patients return for six-month follow-up, 180 complete examinations were performed for every tumor discovered (18) in the thermography-positive group. In our initial screening of the entire population, one tumor was discovered every 100 examinations (10.4/1000). Therefore, rescreening of the thermography-positive group was not as efficient in tumor discovery as would be examining a new unscreened population. If there were 20% additional cancers in the positive-thermogram group as originally projected in our protocol, then the number of examinations necessary for each tumor discovered in this group would have been significantly lower (78) than our normal initial screening experience and would have been of benefit.

Modality Screening Sensitivity and Specificity. The relative sensitivity and specificity for each examining modality will vary according to the definition of what constitutes a positive outcome of the screening test and whether interval cancers that were discovered without a positive examination are included in the diseased category.

The thermographic interpreters were allowed only two decision criteria in their interpretation, i.e. normal (two-year follow-up) or abnormal (early recall). This was not the case for the clinical examiners or the x-ray mammographic interpreters. They were allowed three decision criteria, i.e. normal (two-year follow-up), abnormal (biopsy recommendation) or suspicious (early recall). Attempting to resolve these different outcomes of the different examinations results in various combinations and permutations of sensitivity and specificity determinations. A further complicating factor is that thermography identified 18 tumor cases with an abnormal call (15 at BDC, 3 outside interval cases), before either clinical or x-ray mammography did the same. It is not certain whether these 18 examinations should be credited solely to thermography. Table 9 summarizes the sensitivity and specificity for each examining modality, using the different criteria as outlined above for positivity and disease state within the population.

As shown in Table 9, thermography's sensitivity (37.7% to 43.3%) and specificity (79.2%) are the lowest of all three examining modalities. These results approximate those of the clinical examination and are significantly better than chance alone in determining the presence or absence of breast carcinoma (P $<10^{-9}$). However, these values preclude the use of thermography, in its present state, as an initial screening examination for breast cancer.

Biopsy Sensitivity and Specificity for Each Modality. Thermography exhibits a significant sensitivity and specificity, 40.9% and 70.4%, respectively (P = .004), for breast cancer in those patients for whom biopsy has been recommended by either clinical examination or x-ray mammography. Its specificity for the 208 biopsy cases is almost double that of the other two examining modalities and its sensitivity is not much less

Table 9. Summary of Screening Sensitivities and Specificities

Modality	Sensitivity Range	Specificity Range	χ^2 Significance
Mammography	62.3-78.4	90.1-98.5	$<10^{-9}$
Clinical	39.7-50.5	93.2-98.4	$<10^{-9}$
Thermography	37.7-43.3	79.2	$<10^{-9}$

Table 10. Biopsy Sensitivity and Specificity of Each Modality
(664 Biopsies)

Modality	True Positive	True Negative	True-Positive Rate	False-Negative Rate	Sensitivity	Specificity	χ^2
Mammography	163	195	38.4	18.8	78.4	42.8	$P < 10^{-9}$
Thermography	85	321	38.6	27.7	40.9	70.4	$P = .004$
Clinical	105	176	27.3	36.9	50.5	38.6	$P = .008$
Total	208	456					

than that of clinical examination. Although mammography's sensitivity and specificity are the highest, thermography's are better than those of clinical examination. This indicates that thermography has a role in determining the outcome of a biopsy recommended by another modality. These results are detailed in Table 10.

Modality Accuracy by Tumor Type. Sixty percent of the biopsies performed in our patient population were done at other insitutions. Four hundred thirty-four of the 456 benign biopsies (95.2%) and 201 of the 208 proven noninterval tumor cases discovered (96.6%) were reviewed by the Breast Diagnostic Center pathologist. He has disagreed on four cases; one patient previously thought to have malignancy was subsequently classified as having benign ductal hyperplasia, and three previously reported benign cases were reclassified as lobular carcinoma in situ. All of the cases of discordant diagnoses were sent out to two additional pathologists for confirmation. The diagnosis of the Center's pathologist was the one entered into the patient's master data file and was used for reporting purposes.

We have classified all tumors into the two standard categories that affect prognosis:

    1.   According to invasive characteristics:
        A. Ductal.
           (a) In situ.
           (b) Microinvasive.
           (c) Invasive.

B. Lobular.
 (a) In situ.
 (b) Invasive.
2. According to size:
 A. One centimeter and under with no nodal metastases.
 B. Over 1 cm with or without nodal metastases.

Table 11 classifies each tumor by pathological type related to the degree of invasiveness at each screening period. A very high incidence of in situ and microinvasive lesions (16.3%) and invasive lesions without nodal metastasis (38%) has been discovered in our patient population, as would be expected in a screening protocol. In addition, there has been a very high incidence of low-grade, tubular-type, invasive ductal carcinomas in our patient population (11.5% of all tumors). Although the frequency of this type of carcinoma has been reported as 1% in routine tumor discovery, in our population over 14% of the invasive ductal carcinomas fall into this category. Review of over 100 cases of breast carcinoma that were detected in our institution during a period concurrent with the Breast Diagnostic Center study reveals that the frequency of this type of

Table 11. Tumor Distribution By Pathological Type at Each Screening Period

Tumor Type	Initial	Interval Early Recall	Biennial	Total Tumors
Ductal				
In situ	15 (9.9%)	5 (16.1%)	1 (4%)	21 (10.1%)
Microinvasive	11 (7.2%)	1 (3.2%)	1 (4%)	13 (6.3%)
Tubular	20 (13.2%)	3 (9.6%)	1 (4%)	24 (11.5%)
Invasive –				
No nodes	51 (33.5%)	14 (45.2%)	11 (44%)	76 (36.5%)
Less than 4 LN	23 (15.1%)	5 (16.1%)	6 (24%)	34 (16.4%)
Disseminated	12 (7.9%)	1 (3.2%)	1 (4%)	14 (6.7%)
No nodes reported	10 (6.6%)	1 (3.2%)	–	11 (5.3%)
Lobular				
In situ	8 (5.3%)	–	1 (4%)	9 (4.3%)
Invasive	2 (1.3%)	1 (3.2%)	3 (12%)	6 (2.9%)
Total	152 (100%)	31 (100%)	25 (100%)	208 (100%)*

*Of this number, 201 were pathologically reviewed.

invasive carcinoma is probably higher (8%) than previously reported. It is not surprising that a screening protocol would discover a greater proportion of slow-growing invasive lesions since there should be a higher percentage of these tumors in asymptomatic women.

Table 12, which details modality accuracy by tumor type on all visits, reveals that thermography and clinical examination are least accurate in identifying the in situ ductal carcinomas and most accurate with the infiltrating ductal variety. Mammography shows its highest performance level for the in situ lesions. If further improvement in thermographic accuracy is to be achieved, it will have to be in better identification of the pre-invasive in situ ductal lesions. This is doubly important, for it is this lesion that has the most favorable prognosis.

These findings are confirmed as shown in Table 13, where the tumors are classified by size and presence or absence of metastasis. With a definition of minimal cancer as a tumor less than 1 cm in size without nodal involvement, mammography demonstrated the highest detection rate for these lesions at all examination intervals. Thermography's rate was constant for all examination intervals and was considerably poorer than mammography's. Clinical examination had the poorest detection rate for these minimal tumors and was unable to identify any of

Table 12. Modality Tumor Detection by Pathological Type — All Visits

Tumor Type	Modality			Total Tumors
	M	T	C	
Ductal				
In situ	20 (95.2%)	7 (33.3%)	3 (14.3%)	21 (10.1%)
Microinvasive	9 (69.2%)	4 (30.8%)	4 (30.8%)	13 (6.3%)
Tubular	23 (95.8%)	11 (45.8%)	7 (29.2%)	24 (11.5%)
Invasive —				
No nodes	54 (71.1%)	30 (39.5%)	40 (52.6%)	76 (36.5%)
Less than 4 LN	26 (76.5%)	15 (44.1%)	25 (73.5%)	34 (16.4%)
Disseminated	11 (78.6%)	8 (57.1%)	13 (92.9%)	14 (6.7%)
No nodes reported	8 (72.7%)	4 (36.4%)	7 (63.6%)	11 (5.3%)
Lobular				
In situ	7 (77.8%)	5 (55.6%)	3 (33.3%)	9 (4.3%)
Invasive	5 (83.3%)	1 (16.7%)	3 (50.0%)	6 (2.9%)
Total	163 (78.4%)	85 (40.9%)	105 (50.5%)	208 (100%)

Table 13. Minimal Cancers Detected at Each Screening Period
by Modality*

	Initial	Early Recall	Biennial	Total
Mammography	53 (83%)	12 (80%)	9 (100%)	74 (84%)
Thermography	25 (39%)	8 (53%)	3 (33%)	36 (41%)
Clinical	20 (31%)	3 (20%)	0 (0%)	23 (26%)
Minimal cancers	64 (42%)	15 (48%)	9 (36%)	88 (42%)
Total cancers	152	31	25	208

*Tumors <1 cm in size without nodal involvement.

them on the biennial screen. It can also be noted from this table that the relative percentage of minimal cancers at each screening period was essentially constant. This would indicate once again that the two-year rescreening interval is too long to detect cancers at their early stage of development, assuming effective detection of all tumors from earlier exams. Almost half of the cancers discovered (42%) in this screening protocol satisfied the minimal criteria, which is twice the rate of that found by nonscreening means.

Conclusions

Evaluation of Results in Relation to Originally Stated Objectives

1. To determine whether thermography and clinical examination could be utilized as an initial screening procedure in lieu of mammography and clinical examination with no significant (10%) decrease in female breast cancer detection.

During the protocol mammography in combination with clinical examination detected 84.2% of the cancers as compared to thermography and clinical examination's 59.1% detection rate, a decrease of 30% if thermography was substituted for mammography. This decrease is significantly greater than the anticipated 10% reduction in cancer detection. In addition, in a true screening protocol it would not be desirable to combine a screening modality with clinical examination. Analysis of data on the 17,543 women indicates that thermography is presently not sufficently sensitive to be a one-to-one substitution for mammography. Thermography's apparent 42.1% true-positve detection rate since the beginning of the project is too low to satisfy this objective alone. Therefore, it appears that thermography in its present state cannot be used as an effective screening tool for the early detection of breast cancer.

2. To determine whether the additon of thermography to an examination consisting of mammography and clinical examination would increase the detection rate by a significant amount (20%).

The 18 additional carcinomas discovered initially by thermography alone increased the detection rate by 7%, significantly lower than the anticipated 20% increase by the addition of this examination.

3. To determine whether thermography could be utilized to identify women with high risk of developing clinically demonstrable cancer of the breast within a time period of up to four years.

The incidence rate of cancers in the thermography-positive group is not significantly different from the anticipated normal incidence rate from the general population. Therefore, it appears that thermography is unable to identify a subpopulation of women with a high risk of developing clinically demonstrable cancer. This original objective was also not satisfied by our results.

Conclusions Unstated in Original Objectives

1. Thermography's sensitivity and specificity are poorest in the small, clinically occult minimal cancers.
2. X-ray mammography is the most effective diagnostic technique for detection of minimal cancers.
3. A two-year interval between screening examinations is too long a period to effectively diagnose incident minimal cancers in the screened population.
4. Mammography's 78.4% sensitivity for breast cancer is not as high as previously reported (about 90%), and its 90% to 98% specificity is also lower than previously reported.

References

1. National Cancer Institute: The Third National Cancer Survey: Incidence Data, DHEW Publication No. (NIH) 75-787, National Institutes of Health, 1975.
2 Adair, F., Berg, J.W., Joubert, L. and Robbins, G.F.: Long term follow-up of breast cancer patients: The 30-year report. Cancer 33 (4):1145-1150, 1974.
3. Haagensen, C.D.: Diseases of the Breast. Philadelphia:W. B Saunders, 1971, p. 706.
4. Pomerance, W., Connor, R.J., Fink, D.J. et al: Screening for breast cancer. Lancet 1:143, 1976.
5. Bailar, J.C.: Mammography: A contrary view. Ann. Intern. Med. 84 (1):77-84, 1976.
6. Barnes, R.B.: Thermography. Ann. N.Y. Acad. Sci. 121:34-48, 1964.
7. Macey, D.J. and Oliver, R.: Image resolution in infrared thermography. Phy. Med. Biol. 17:563-571, 1972.
8. Wolfe, W.L.: Infrared imaging devices in infrared medical radiography. Ann. N.Y. Acad. Sci. 121:57-70, 1964.
9. Watmough, D.J. and Oliver, R.: Wavelength dependence of skin emissivity. Phys. Med. Biol. 14:201-204, 1969.
10. Hardy, J.D.: Radiating power of human skin in infrared. Am. J. Physiol. 127:454, 1939.
11. Watmough, D.J. and Oliver, R.: The emission of infrared radiation from human skin — Implications for clinical thermography. Br. J. Radiol. 42:411-415, 1969.
12. Dreyfus, M.G.: Spectral variations of black body radiation. Appl. Optics 2:1113, 1963.
13. Fay, T. and Henry, G.C.: Correlation of body segmental temperature and its relation to the location of carcinomatous metastases. Surg. Gynecol. Obstet. 66:512-524, 1938.
14. Lawson, R.N.: Implication of surface temperatures in the diagnosis of breast cancer. Can. Med. Assoc. J. 75:309-310, 1956.
15. Lawson, R.N. and Shughtai, M.S.: Breast cancer and body temperature. Can. Med. Assoc. J. 88:68-70, 1963.
16. Lloyd-Williams, K., Lloyd-Williams, F.J. and Handley, R.S.: Infrared thermography in the diagnosis of breast disease. Lancet 2:1378-1381, 1961.
17. Lawson, R.N. and Gaston, J.P.: Temperature measurements of localized pathologic processes. Ann. N.Y. Acad. Sci. 121:90-98, 1964.
18. Dodd, G.D., Zermeno, A., Wallace, J.D. and Marsh, L.: Breast thermography: The state of the art. Curr. Probl. Radiol. 3:6, 1973.
19. Davy, J.B., Greening, W.P. and McKinna, J.A.: Is screening of cancer worthwhile? Results from a well-woman clinic for cancer detection. Br. Med. J. 3:696, 1970.
20. Isard, H.J., Ostrum, B.J. and Shilo, R.: Thermography in breast carcinoma. Surg. Gynecol. Obstet. 128:1289, 1969.

21. Stark, A.M. and Way, S.: Screening for breast cancer. Lancet 2:407, 1970.
22. Dowdy, A.H., Lagasse, L.D., Sperling, L. et al: A combined screening program for the detection of carcinoma of the cervix and carcinoma of the breast. Surg. Gynecol. Obstet. 131:93, 1970.
23. Tricoire, J., Mariel, L., Amiel, J.P. et al: Thermographie en plaque. Presse Med. 55:2483, 1970.
24. Dodd, G.D., Wallace, J.D., Freundlich, I.M. et al: Thermography and cancer of the breast. Cancer 23:797, 1969.
25. Isard, H.J., Becker, W., Shilo, R. and Ostrum, B.J.: Breast thermography after four years and 10,000 studies. Am. J. Roentgenol. 115:811, 1972.
26. Furnival, I.G., Stewart, H.J., Wedell, J.M. et al: Accuracy of screening methods for the diagnosis of breast disease. Br. Med. J. 4:461, 1970.

Self-Evaluation Quiz

1. A two-year interval between screening examination appears to be too long for detection of small incident carcinomas.
   a) True
   b) False
2. In this study, the effectiveness of mammography and clinical examination in identifying tumors decreased on the early recall examination but rose for both on the two-year follow-up.
   a) True
   b) False
3. Thermography showed significant effectiveness on early recall, but not on biennial examination.
   a) True
   b) False
4. Thermography's sensitivity and specificity were poorest in the small, clinically occult minimal cancers.
   a) True
   b) False
5. Thermography and clinical examination were least accurate in identifying ___ and most accurate for ___ ; mammography was most accurate for ___ .
   a) In situ lesions
   b) In situ ductal carcinomas
   c) Infiltrating ductal carcinomas

Answers on page 335.

Breast Cancer and Exogenous Estrogens: The Epidemiologic Evidence

Barbara S. Hulka, M.D., M.P.H.

Objectives

1. To summarize the results from the published epidemiologic literature which have attempted to demonstrate an association between exogenous estrogen use and breast cancer.
2. To present these results in such a way that they may be evaluated by clinicians and viewed in conjunction with the existing clinical, pathologic and endocrinologic data.

Breast cancer is the number one cause of cancer deaths among women in the United States [1]. Over 33,000 deaths from breast cancer occurred in 1976 and over 100,000 new cases were estimated for 1979. Age-adjusted mortality rates for white women in the United States have remained fairly constant at about 25 per 100,000 per year from 1935 to 1974 [2]. For non-white women, mortality rates were lower in the early period, but they rose to rates almost as high as those for white women in 1973 to 1974. Incidence rates reported from the U.S. National Cancer Surveys have also remained fairly constant for whites but have increased for non-whites. In contrast to the U.S. National Cancer Surveys, data from Alberta, Canada, show a steady increase in incidence of about 1 per 100,000 women per year between 1953 and 1973 [3]. Also, an increasing incidence has been noted in England and Wales, as well as from

Barbara S. Hulka, M.D., M.P.H., Professor, Department of Epidemiology, University of North Carolina, Chapel Hill.

the Connecticut Tumor Registry in the United States [4]. The increase has been most prominent since the mid-1960s among women over age 45. Although various explanations for these increases have been set forth, such as alterations in fertility and diet, none seem to be well substantiated. Since the increases are temporally associated with increases in estrogen prescribing [5], a more direct association between these two phenomena has been sought in a large number of epidemiologic studies. Some of the more recent studies are summarized in Tables 1 and 2.

The eight case-control studies shown in Table 1 provide very little support for an association between estrogen use and breast cancer. The study of Wynder et al [6] included a large number of pre-, peri- and post-menopausal patients and controls. Each of the three menopausal categories was analyzed separately, and no excess estrogen use was found for any of the case groups. Among postmenopausal women, 6.0% of cases and 9.7% of controls had used estrogens for 20 months or more. Data were not presented for longer periods of use.

Table 1. Case-Control Studies of Exogenous Estrogen and Breast Cancer

First Author	Cases Yr. of Dx	No.	Controls Source	No.	Relative Risk*
Wynder [6]	1969-75	785	Hospital	2231	1.1
Sartwell [7]	1969-72	284	Hospital	367	0.8
Boston Collaborative Drug Surveillance Program [8]	1972	51	Hospital	774	1.0
Brinton [13]	1973-77	405	Screening program	1156	1.0
Henderson [12]	1969-72	308	Physicians' offices	308	0.8
Casagrande [9]	1972-73	47	Neighborhood	31	3.1
Craig [10]	1949-67	134	Population & neighborhood	260	1.0
Mack [11]	1971-75	111	Community	444	1.6

*Relative risk is for "ever use" of estrogen.

The Sartwell [7] study was designed specifically to evaluate the effect of estrogens and oral contraceptives on breast cancer risk. No positive association was found in any analysis. Estrogen use for five years or more produced a relative risk (RR) for breast cancer of 0.6, suggesting no excess risk and possibly a protective effect from estrogen. The results of the Boston Collaborative Drug Surveillance Program [8] confirmed the lack of increased risk.

The Casagrande [9] study produced an apparent increased risk of 3.1, but with only 47 cases and 31 controls, this result was not statistically significant. The data from Craig et al [10] showed no increased risk, but the question about use of "female hormones" was not sufficiently specific to obtain reliable information on estrogen use. Mack et al [11] focused on the possible association between reserpine and breast cancer, and medical record data were collected about different types of prescribed medications. Breast cancer risk was slightly, although not significantly, elevated for several medications, including antihypertensives, thiazides, barbiturates and estrogens. These results do not incriminate any particular medication but do suggest that women who are prone to use medical services also may be prone to develop breast cancer.

Henderson et al [12] made the observation that women using estrogens for menopausal symptoms were at reduced breast cancer risk during the first nine postmenopausal years (RR = 0.2). During the subsequent postmenopausal years, this protective effect was lost (RR = 1.7). These findings were based on 94 patients and 83 controls who had undergone a natural menopause. The authors conclude that "exogenous hormones are clearly associated with a reduced risk of breast cancer."

The large study by Brinton et al [13] demonstrated no association between estrogen and breast cancer, even after long durations of use (15 years or more). All relative risks were unity or less, except for risks associated with five to nine years' duration of use or five to nine years since first use. For these categories, the relative risks were 1.8 and 1.6, respectively, although the lower boundary of the 95% confidence interval for each relative risk included unity.

Table 2 summarizes the follow-up studies, in which subjects were identified retrospectively through private practice or clinic

Table 2. Practice-Based Follow-up Studies of Exogenous Estrogen
and Breast Cancer

First Author	Number Estrogen Exposed	Number Not Estrogen Exposed	Intake and Follow-up Period	Definition of Estrogen Use	Relative Risk
Byrd [14]	1016 (33)*	0	1948-76	>3 yr	1.4
Hoover [15]	1891 (49)	0	1939-72	≥6 mo	1.3
Hammond [16]	301 (4)	309 (4)	1940-75	≥5 yr	1.1

*Numbers of incident breast cancer cases are in parentheses.

records and then followed prospectively to identify their subsequent morbidity and mortality. In the Byrd et al study [14], hysterectomized women attending a single practice in Nashville, Tennessee, were prescribed estrogens and followed for 5 to 28 years. Expected numbers of incident breast cancer cases were obtained from the Third National Cancer Survey, based on the Atlanta, Georgia, experience. Breast cancer incidence was excessive (relative risks about 4.0) for estrogen use of less than ten years' duration. The increased risks were particularly notable for nulliparous women. Risks dropped to about unity after ten years or more of estrogen use. Expected numbers of deaths were obtained from vital statistics in the state of Tennessee. No excess mortality from breast cancer has occurred in the estrogen-exposed cohort: six deaths observed and eight expected.

The Hoover et al [15] study was also based on a cohort of women using estrogen, many of whom had had hysterectomy and all of whom came from a single practice in Louisville, Kentucky. No early increase in breast cancer risk was demonstrated. Rather, a statistically significant increased risk of 2.0 appeared only after 15 years of follow-up. Duration of estrogen use was highly correlated with duration of follow-up, and no independent effect of duration was found. The inconsistent results from the Byrd et al and Hoover et al follow-up studies are not readily explainable. In both studies, Third National Cancer Survey data were used to formulate the expected number of breast cancer cases. To what extent these expected numbers are relevant to women in the individual practices is not known.

Hammond et al [16] used a cohort approach including both estrogen-exposed and estrogen-unexposed women. However, the numbers in each group were small, and the two groups differed on demographic characteristics and clinical features at the time of entry into the study.

Summary

The preponderance of evidence from well-designed, case-control studies shows no increased risk of breast cancer associated with use of exogenous estrogen. These studies were done in different regions of the United States and included large numbers of subjects. Cases were obtained from hospitals, tumor registries and defined populations. Likewise, the control series were drawn from diverse sources, usually corresponding to those of the cases. If a decisive breast cancer risk due to estrogen existed, it should have been manifest through these multiple studies.

Two follow-up studies of estrogen-exposed women produced divergent results; one suggested an increased risk with less than ten years of estrogen use and no increased risk thereafter, and the other reported an increased risk only after 15 years of use. These conflicting results require reconciliation before a firm statement on the relationship of exogenous estrogen to breast cancer can be made. Breast tissue is hormonally dependent, and it is not unreasonable to suppose that exogenous as well as endogenous estrogen would have an effect upon it. Epidemiologic studies alone have not been able to characterize this effect.

References

1. Cancer Statistics, 1979. Based on data from the National Cancer Institute's Surveillance, Epidemiology and End Results (SEER) Program (1973-1976). CA 29 (1):6-21, 1979.
2. Devesa, S.S. and Silverman, D.T.: Cancer incidence and mortality trends in the United States: 1935-74. JNCI 60 (3):545-571, 1978.
3. Grace, M., Gaudette, L.A. and Burns, P.E.: The increasing incidence of breast cancer in Alberta, 1953-1973. Cancer 40 (1):358-363, 1977.
4. Armstrong, B.: Recent trends in breast-cancer incidence and mortality in relation to changes in possible risk factors. Int. J. Cancer 17:204-211, 1976.

5. Current Industrial Reports: Pharmaceutical Preparations, Except Biologicals, 1974, Series: MA-28G(74)-1. U.S. Department of Commerce, Bureau of Census, 1975.
6. Wynder, E.L., MacCormack, F.A. and Stellman, S.D.: The epidemiology of breast cancer in 785 United States Caucasian women. Cancer 41 (6):2341-2354, 1978.
7. Sartwell, P.E., Arthes, F.G. and Tonascia, J.A.: Exogenous hormones, reproductive history, and breast cancer. JNCI 59 (6):1589-1592, 1977.
8. Boston Collaborative Drug Surveillance Program, Boston University Medical Center: Surgically confirmed gallbladder disease, venous thromboembolism and breast tumors in relation to postmenopausal estrogen therapy. N. Engl. J. Med. 290 (1):15-19, 1974.
9. Casagrande, J., Gerkins, V., Henderson, B.E. et al: Brief communication: Exogenous estrogens and breast cancer in women with natural menopause. JNCI 56 (4):839-841, 1976.
10. Craig, T.J., Comstock, G.W. and Geiser, P.B.: Epidemiologic comparison of breast cancer patients with early and late onset of malignancy and general population controls. JNCI 53 (6):1577-1581, 1974.
11. Mack, T.M., Henderson, B.E., Gerkins, V.R. et al: Reserpine and breast cancer in a retirement community. N. Engl. J. Med. 292 (26):1366-1371, 1975.
12. Henderson, B.E., Powell, D., Rosario, I. et al: An epidemiologic study of breast cancer. JNCI 53 (3):609-614, 1974.
13. Brinton, L.A., Williams, R.R., Hoover, R.N. et al: Breast cancer risk factors among screening program participants. JNCI 62 (1):37-44, 1979.
14. Byrd, B.F., Burch, J.C. and Vaughn, W.K.: The impact of long term estrogen support after hysterectomy, a report of 1016 cases. Ann. Surg. 185 (5):574-580, 1977.
15. Hoover, R., Gray, L.A., Cole, P. and MacMahon, B.: Menopausal estrogens and breast cancer. N. Engl. J. Med. 295 (8):401-405, 1976.
16. Hammond, C.B., Jelovsek, F.R., Lee, K.L. et al: Effects of long-term estrogen replacement therapy: II. Neoplasia. Am. J. Obstet. Gynecol. 133 (5):537-547, 1979.

The material in this paper is excerpted from Hulka, B.S.: Effect of exogenous estrogen on postmenopausal women: The epidemiologic evidence. Obstet. Gynecol. Surv. 35 (suppl. 6):389-399, 1980. Copyright 1980, The Williams and Wilkins Co., Baltimore.

Self-Evaluation Quiz

1. The summary relative risks as reported in eight case-control studies published in the 1970s demonstrated no statistically significant association between estrogen use and breast cancer.
    a) True
    b) False

2. Which of the following is correct concerning two practice-based follow-up studies that produced divergent results?
    a) The Byrd et al study (Nashville, Tenn.) showed no increased breast cancer risk, but the Hoover et al study (Louisville, Ky.) showed a greatly increased breast cancer risk following estrogen use
    b) The Byrd et al study showed an increased breast cancer risk during the first ten postmenopausal years and the Hoover et al study showed an increased breast cancer risk after 15 years of estrogen use
    c) Neither of the above

3. Case-control studies:
    a) Compare the proportion of women with breast cancer who have been exposed to estrogens with the proportion of non-cases (controls) who have been exposed to estrogen
    b) Compare the proportion of estrogen users who develop breast cancer with the proportion of nonusers who develop breast cancer
    c) Neither of the above

4. Follow-up studies of women exposed to estrogen are subject to a number of methodologic constraints. Which of the following methodologic constraints are characteristic of follow-up studies?
    a) Expected numbers of women getting the disease (breast cancer) have to be obtained from some source, and women from that source may or may not be comparable to the women in the group being followed
    b) Large numbers of estrogen-exposed women are required in order to generate a meaningful number of breast cancer cases even after many years of follow-up

   c) If many women are "lost to follow-up," confidence in the results of the study is lessened

   d) All of the above

5. Considering the published epidemiologic data on breast cancer and estrogens, along with the existing biological and clinical data, which of the following statements is most likely to be true?

   a) Exogenous estrogens taken for menopausal symptoms cause breast cancer

   b) Breast tissue is hormonally dependent and is influenced by either exogenous or endogenous estrogens, but a causative role of estrogens in relation to breast cancer has not been established

   c) Neither of the above

Answers on page 335.

The Selective Surgical Treatment of Potentially Curable Breast Cancer

Henry Patrick Leis, Jr., M.D.

Objectives

1. To emphasize the magnitude of the breast cancer problem and the importance of the surgeon's role in its management.
2. To describe the various types of surgical procedures used and to discuss the changing picture from radical to lesser types of operations.
3. To present current evaluation studies by the NSABP, the criteria used for selecting various surgical procedures, the major types of selective surgical approaches, the role of primary radiotherapy, the NIH Consensus Conference recommendations and the importance of obtaining hormone receptor studies.
4. To present a moderate selective surgical approach for patients with potentially curable breast cancers, with the results obtained in 846 patients followed for ten or more years as to survival and local recurrence rates and cosmetic and functional results, and to compare these results with those from other types of surgical approaches and from primary radiotherapy.
5. To present a rational approach to the management of the other breast and to discuss breast reconstruction in properly selected patients.

Introduction

The magnitude of the breast cancer problem is emphasized by the fact that it is the most common cancer in women,

Henry Patrick Leis, Jr., M.D., F.A.C.S., F.I.C.S. (Hon.), Clinical Professor of Surgery; Chief of Breast Service; Co-Director, Institute of Breast Diseases, New York Medical College, Valhalla, N.Y.; Chief of Breast Surgery, Cabrini Medical Center, New York City.

accounting for about 28% of all the cancers that develop in them. One out of every 11 women, or about 9%, will develop breast cancer during her lifetime. In 1979, in the United States alone, there were about 106,900 new cases [1].

Once the diagnosis of cancer and its exact nature have been established by biopsy and histologic examination [2] and the necessary preoperative work-up has been completed [3], then consideration must be given to the selection of the most appropriate surgical procedure, to the proper management of the other breast and to the possibility of performing restorative surgery.

Surgeon's Role in Breast Cancer

Even if one accepts some of the postulates of Fisher [4, 5] — i.e., that all breast cancers are systemic at their time of onset, that regional nodes are not a barrier to the dissemination of tumor cells, and that their removal does not influence survival rates — the surgeon's position in the care of the breast cancer patient is still one of *prime* importance.

The surgeon removes the tumor load rapidly, without causing immunosuppression. He provides for pathologic staging by removal of the axillary nodes. He removes tissue that can be used for testing the immunocompetence of the host at the time of surgery and afterward [6, 7], for doing estrogen and progesterone receptor studies [8, 9] and for histologic studies regarding the tumor growth potential or virulence — all of which can be used in determining the patient's prognosis and need for adjuvant therapy [10-13]. Finally, he offers the patient a high likelihood for local and regional control [14-17] of her cancer and lays the groundwork for possible systemic therapy without a long period of delay.

Surgical Procedures

There are a number of operations that have been recommended for patients with potentially curable breast cancers, including tumorectomy or lumpectomy; tylectomy; partial or segmental mastectomy; subcutaneous mastectomy; simple, or total or complete mastectomy; limited or conservative modified radical mastectomy; full modified radical mastectomy; radical mastectomy; and extended radical mastectomy.

1. *Segmental or partial mastectomy*, which entails removal of one quarter to one third of the breast with the overlying skin [18-20], can be accompanied by an axillary node sampling or an axillary gland dissection [21]. In tylectomy the skin does not have to be removed, and tumorectomy or lumpectomy refers to just removal of the tumor.

2. *Subcutaneous mastectomy or adenomammectomy* is a procedure in which the breast tissue is shelled out as completely as possible, with preservation of the skin, nipple and areola [22].

3. In a *simple, total or complete mastectomy*, the entire breast is removed and in most centers an axillary node sampling is done. Our average node count in this operation was 7.8.

4. In the *conservative or limited type of modified radical mastectomy*, the entire breast is removed and there is a thorough and careful dissection of the first level of axillary nodes. Most surgeons start the dissection at the lateral border of the pectoralis minor muscle and preserve both pectoral muscles, as well as the second or pectoral level and the third or superior apical level of nodes.

In our technique [14-16], the pectoralis minor muscle is routinely retracted, and we remove part or all of the second level of nodes and carefully palpate the superior apical and interpectoral node areas. With this technique our average node count was 22.3.

Some authorities, like Auchincloss [23], Caceras [24] and Madden [25], attempt to remove all three levels of nodes, with or without severance of the pectoralis minor muscle near its insertion into the coracoid process. Kodama [26] splits the sulcus interpectoralis between the clavicular and sternocostal heads of the pectoralis major muscle, and then severs the pectoralis minor muscle near its insertion and does a resection of all three levels of nodes. Schmitz [27], in an attempt to better obliterate the axillary space and avoid dog-ears at the wound extremities, removes triangular sections of excess skin in the center of both flaps, but this results in a cross-shaped wound.

5. The *full, total or complete type of modified radical mastectomy*, as first described by Patey [28] and popularized by Handley [29], removes all the structures that are resected in the classical radical, except for the pectoralis major muscle.

It is a more difficult and time-consuming procedure to perform than the classical radical. Great care must be used not to injure the nerve and blood supply to the pectoralis major muscle; otherwise, it will atrophy and give an appearance similar to that of the radical mastectomy. Our average node count with this type of modified radical mastectomy was 31.9.

Roses, Harris and Gumport [30] modified this type of operation by dividing the pectoralis major muscle between its clavicular and sternal portions, with care to preserve its blood and nerve supply. They felt that this facilitated the dissection of the nodes, especially at the apex. After the dissection is completed they reconstruct the muscle.

6. The *standard radical mastectomy*, as first described by Halsted [31], entails removal of the entire breast, both pectoral muscles, Rotter's interpectoral nodes, the deep pectoral fascia with all three levels of nodes and the subcapsular fascia with the subcapular nodes. Our average node count with the standard radical mastectomy was 32.2.

7. In the *extended radical mastectomy* [32], for which there are a number of modifications, the internal mammary nodes are removed in addition to the standard radical mastectomy procedure.

Procedure Evaluation Studies

In an attempt to evaluate the value of various methods of breast cancer treatment, the National Surgical Adjuvant Breast Project (NSABP) was organized in 1957 by the National Cancer Institute. Since it was believed that an answer could *not* be obtained from historical data — no matter how detailed or how carefully analyzed — but only by randomized, prospective, controlled clinical trials, a project was started in the fall of 1971 with investigators from 34 institutions in the United States and Canada [4]. They agreed to participate in a protocol comparing alternative treatments of primary operable breast cancer with radical mastectomy. Women were randomized into three therapy groups: radical mastectomy, total mastectomy and total mastectomy with regional radiotherapy. Those patients with clinically positive axillary nodes were randomly assigned to either radical mastectomy or total mastectomy with regional irradiation. To date the findings are only provisional, but in those patients followed for six years, no significant difference has been noted in the various groups. The problem with these trials is that they are not really randomized because of patient and physician selection, lack of participation and patient withdrawal. Questions have also been raised regarding whether all the procedures were done with equal detail and completeness, and whether adjuvant therapy was at variance in some selected patients.

The NSABP has recently implemented another protocol to see whether cosmetically acceptable preservation of the breast, in a subset of patients with primary cancer, can be achieved without unfavorably influencing treatment failure and survival rates [4]. Appropriate patients who are eligible for segmental mastectomy, as defined in the protocol, following stratification according to nodal status and tumor size, are randomized into three groups. They are treated by either total mastectomy and axillary dissection, segmental mastectomy and axillary dissection, or segmental mastectomy and axillary dissection, followed by irradiation to the breast. Patients in all three groups who have histologically positive axillary nodes receive adjuvant chemotherapy. Since the trial only began in 1976, no statistically valuable data are available yet.

Many major medical centers feel strongly that no one operation or procedure is applicable to, or best for, every patient with breast cancer, and that there are enough historical, statistically well-documented data with adequate criteria for efficacy evaluation to enable a surgeon to select a specific type of operation for each patient. The aim is to tailor the operation to fit each situation, offering a maximum of benefit with a minimum of trauma. The primary goal, however, must always be cure; cosmetic appearance and functional results must be subservient to this.

Criteria For Procedure Selection

The choice of procedure to be used is based on a number of criteria [10-13, 15, 16], including:

1. The anatomic extent of the cancer (i.e. its stage, size and location).
2. Its growth potential or virulence (i.e. its invasiveness, multicentricity, histologic type, grade or degree of

cellular differentiation, growth pattern, central necrosis, and lymphatic permeation and blood vessel invasion into surrounding tissue).
3. The patient's age and constitutional status.

In some centers, including ours at New York Medical College, tests are performed to measure the immunologic resistance of the host, at the time of surgery and following it [6, 7]. These tests are used in evaluating the patient's prognosis and in helping to determine the advisability of using adjuvant therapy after surgery.

Selective Surgical Approaches

While many centers agree that surgery should be performed on a selective basis, there is a difference of opinion as to which operations should be employed in the selective approach. In general, there seem to be three main types of selective surgical approaches, i.e. conservative, radical and moderate.

The types of mastectomy utilized in the conservative approach, as reported by Crile [18] and Hermann [19, 20] from the Cleveland Clinic, are (1) segmental or partial, (2) simple or total, and (3) limited modified radical. An attempt is made to preserve the regional lymph nodes, when possible, with the belief that they may act as repositories of systemic immunity preventing the distant spread of cancer. It is postulated that all breast tissue need not be removed in small, peripherally located cancers if there is little likelihood of multicentricity, and that muscles should not be sacrificed. The majority of operations performed at Cleveland Clinic are limited modified radical mastectomies.

The radical approach, as reported by Urban [32] from the Memorial Sloan-Kettering Cancer Center, utilized the following types of mastectomy: (1) limited modified radical, (2) full modified radical, (3) radical, and (4) extended radical. The belief is that all breast tissue should always be removed, as well as one or both pectoral muscles and one or all three levels of axillary nodes, and the internal mammary nodes if there is a strong likelihood that they might be involved. The majority of operations performed at Memorial Hospital are radical mastectomies.

The types of mastectomy utilized in the moderate approach, as recommended by Leis from New York Medical College [14-16], are (1) simple or total, (2) limited modified radical, (3) full modified radical, and (4) radical. The premise is that all breast tissue should be removed but that muscles as well as regional nodes should not be sacrificed unnecessarily, and that central and medial lesions can be treated just as well by adjuvant radiotherapy to the internal mammary nodes as by extended radical mastectomy. The full modified (Patey) radical mastectomy is the most commonly used procedure.

Few centers utilize partial or segmental mastectomies or subcutaneous mastectomies because of the multicentricity of breast cancer, as unequivocally demonstrated in studies by Gallager and Martin [33] and by Rosen and his associates [34]. While admitting that multicentric foci of cancer are often present, Crile [18] and Fisher [4, 5] feel that the development of new clinical cancers in any remaining breast tissue is infrequent. It is also important to note that, despite the cosmetic triumphs that have been credited to segmental mastectomies, the results often leave much to be desired.

At the National Institutes of Health Consensus Conference on "The Treatment of Primary Breast Cancer: Management of Local Disease" held on June 5, 1979 [21], it was the consensus of the panel to support further clinical investigation into the role of segmental mastectomy in the treatment of primary breast cancer.

Only a small number of centers advise extended radical mastectomies — even in central and medial lesions where the possibility of internal mammary node metastases is increased — because of the increased morbidity, poor patient acceptance and a lack of clear-cut evidence, in most centers, of statistically significant improvement in survival rates.

Change in Surgical Procedure Popularity

For many years the classic radical mastectomy, as described by Halsted [31], was the operation of choice for patients with invasive, potentially curable breast cancers. Recently, due in part to earlier diagnosis and to the increasing awareness of physicians and the lay public that properly selected lesser operations can offer comparable survival and recurrence rates, there has been a distinct shift toward operations of less magnitude. In the United States the most popular operation is now the modified radical mastectomy [17, 35].

At the American College of Surgeons Congress in 1974, I presented my results with the selective use of different types of modified radical mastectomies, which I have been using with increasing frequency since 1950. Afterward, the moderator of the panel asked for a show of hands of those who preferred the radical mastectomy to the modified proceduress. The majority of surgeons in the audience raised their hands in support of the classic radical [36].

Between 1960 and 1967, only about 11% of patients with breast cancers underwent a modified radical mastectomy. In 1972 the Breast Cancer Survey of the Commission on Cancer of the American College of Surgeons reported that the classic radical mastectomy was done in 50% of patients and the modified radical in 30% [35]. But in 1977 the Commission reported that the figures were reversed, with 63% of the patients having a modified radical mastectomy while only 22% had a classic radical operation [35]. Today, in most major teaching centers the percentage use of the modified radical mastectomy is even higher [4, 14-21, 25, 29, 30, 37-40].

Unfortunately, there is a wide variance in what is meant by a modified radical mastectomy; some surgeons use the term when they do little more than a simple mastectomy with axillary sampling. At the 1979 NIH Consensus Conference [21], the panel agreed that a procedure that preserves the pectoral muscles, i.e. a total mastectomy with axillary dissection, should be recognized as the current treatment standard for women who have stage I and *selected* stage II breast cancers.

Primary Radiotherapy

Recently, there has been a rapidly growing interest in an approach utilizing limited surgery with irradiation as a primary form of therapy [41-51]. The limited surgery varies from simply a tumorectomy, to a tylectomy, to a segmental mastectomy, with or without axillary sampling or full dissection. This technique, aimed at preserving the breast, has been used for many years at the Foundation Curie in France [44], and now some centers in the United States and Canada are utilizing it [51]. The NIH Consensus Conference also supported further clinical investigations into the role of radiotherapy as a form of primary therapy [21]. It offers an alternative or second choice to patients who are adamantly opposed to having their breast removed.

Reports of treatment failures, early and late complications and survival rates are at considerable variance [51]. Concern is being expressed in many centers regarding delayed radiation effects, including radiation-induced cancers in the breast itself, despite the low incidence of radiation-induced cancers in the regional areas beyond the breast or in the chest wall in the past. The proof of the postulate that all breast tissue is destroyed by large radiation doses so that radiation-induced breast cancers will not occur, must await a prolonged period of follow-up. It is mandatory that large series, with strict criteria for evaluation [12] and with long-term follow-ups, be available for study before conclusions are drawn as to the efficacy of this approach.

Value of Established Procedures

A great deal of reservation has been expressed in a number of major medical centers about the trend away from procedures which have proved their efficacy over a long period of time and toward unproven modalities which, in the long run, may prove to be detrimental to the patient. They feel that unproven procedures should be limited to carefully controlled protocols in selected centers and not tried on the general population.

Hormone Receptors

Estrogen and progesterone receptor studies [8, 9] should be done routinely on all patients with breast cancers when there is adequate tissue. With these tests it is possible to determine whether the cancer is probably hormone dependent so that appropriate hormonal manipulations can be utilized if indicated.

Moderate Selective Surgical Approach

In our moderate selective surgical approach, patients are divided into different groups, with an appropriate operation selected for each one [4, 5, 52].

In the *first group* are patients with noninvasive cancers. They are treated by simple mastectomy with axillary sampling, with an average node count of 7.8. Of the two types of noninvasive cancers, i.e. intraductal and lobular in situ, the latter is usually multicentric and commonly bilateral; therefore, bilateral simple mastectomies are advised. These patients are excellent candidates for restorative procedures.

The *second group* includes patients over 70 years of age, except for those who are in very good health and thus are able to tolerate more extensive surgery, if it is indicated; those with severe constitutional diseases; and those with sarcomas which metastasize predominantly through the blood stream. These patients are treated by simple mastectomy and axillary sampling.

Patients with preclinical invasive cancers, smaller than the 1-cm size that is usually needed for clinical palpation, make up the *third group*. These are treated by a limited or conservative radical mastectomy. Nine of our 58 patients with preclinical invasive cancers, or 15.5%, had positive nodes, but these were usually minimal and confined to the lower axillary nodes. Our average node count was 22.3.

During the past ten years we have employed an increasing number of conservative types of modified radical mastectomies. They are used in patients with good prognostic cancers that are less than 2 cm in pathologic size, and in those who have no evidence of involvement of their second and third levels of axillary nodes or of Rotter's nodes by palpation during surgery. We are now doing more conservative modified mastectomies than full types, and our percentage of classic radical mastectomies is now less than 5%.

The *fourth group* includes patients with invasive cancers of a histologic type that is not prone to metastasize and has a good prognosis, including adenoid cystic, colloid, comedo with minimal stromal invasion, medullary with lymphoid infiltrate, papillary and tubular. These are treated by a full modified radical mastectomy, with an average node count of 31.9.

Patients with other invasive cancers, including the common "no special type," or scirrhous, and the uncommon invasive lobular, make up the *fifth group*. In the past only about 70% of these patients were treated by the full modified radical mastectomy, but now this percentage is much higher. The radical mastectomy was reserved for patients with cancers larger than 3 cm in pathologic measurement; for those whose cancer was close to or apparently involved the pectoralis major muscle, or very near to the sternum or clavicle; and for those with an apparent involvement of Rotter's nodes. The average node count with the radical mastectomy was 32.2.

In both the conservative and full modified radical mastectomy, if the lesion is close to the pectoralis major muscle with possible involvement of it, we now remove a portion of the muscle in the area of concern.

In the *sixth group* of patients with inflammatory cancers, surgery is confined to biopsy and therapy is with radiation, hormones and chemicals.

Management of the Remaining Breast

When definitive breast cancer surgery is performed, attention must be paid to the other breast since it is truly an organ at risk. We do a random biopsy on it, whenever possible, at the time of definitive surgery on the first breast. If a cancer is found, appropriate therapy is instituted. If not, the patient is followed very carefully. Only if she is in the high-risk group for developing cancer in the remaining breast is prophylactic removal by simple mastectomy advised [53, 54].

This high-risk group [53, 54] includes patients whose initial cancer in the first breast carried a good prognosis for extended survival, and whose age and constitutional status do not exclude at least a 20-year normal life expectancy. Thus patients under 50 years of age, in good health, with early cancers (stages 0 and I) that are either noninvasive or of a good prognostic type if invasive, have a high risk for developing cancer in the second breast.

Also included are patients who have special features that indicate an increased risk for bilaterality, such as those with a close family history of breast cancer [55, 56], those whose cancers in the first breast were multicentric, and those who had evidence of precancerous mastopathy [57] in the random biopsy of their other breast [53, 54].

Finally, those patients whose other breast shows a DY (dense parenchymal) pattern on x-ray [58] and those with abnormal thermograms [59] of their remaining breast must be considered at high risk.

Restorative Surgery

While the indications, timing and techniques are still open to debate, there is an ever increasing interest on the part of physicians and patients alike in breast reconstructions after mastectomy [16, 60-64]. At the time of doing a mastectomy we plan on the possibility of doing restorative surgery, as long as this does not jeopardize the patient's chance for cure. Efforts are made to use transverse or oblique incisions, to preserve the pectoralis major muscle and to avoid skin grafting and chest wall kilovoltage (orthovoltage) radiotherapy.

Some centers feel that any patient who wants restorative surgery should be entitled to it. We feel that it is not advisable for every postmastectomy patient and reserve it for those who have a good prognosis for cure, who have little likelihood of local recurrence, and who have not had skin grafts or chest wall kilovoltage radiotherapy. With supervoltage radiotherapy, re-construction is usually possible. A few centers are doing immediate reconstructions, but we wait at least six months to a year to ensure adequate vascularization and loosening of the flaps, and also to allow adequate time for thorough prognostic evaluation.

Results with Moderate Selective Approach

Data were collected for a series of 2,164 patients with primary breast cancers treated at New York Medical College Affiliated Hospitals (1950-1977). The absolute (no evidence of disease) survival rates by stages for 846 patients with potentially curable breast cancers followed for ten or more years are summarized in Table 1. Of the 846 patients, 779 (92.1%) had invasive cancers and their survival rate was 59.9%; 680 (80.3%) of these patients had less than a radical mastectomy. The most commonly used operation was the full modified radical mastec-tomy, which was employed in 564 patients (66.7%).

Table 1. Absolute Ten-Year Survival Rates in
846 Patients
(Stages 0, I and II)

	No. Survivors/ Total No. Patients	%
Stage 0	112/116	96.5
Noninvasive	66/67	98.5
Invasive	46/49	93.9
Stage I	287/397	72.2
Stage II	134/333	40.2
Stages I and II	421/730	57.6
Stages 0, 1 and II	533/846	63.0

The ten-year local recurrence rates in these 846 patients are summarized in Table 2.

Staging

The staging system that we use for patients with potentially curable breast cancers, both clinical and pathological, is a simple three-stage classification (stages 0, I and II) that correlates easily with the more detailed TNM classification (Table 3) [65].

Table 2. Local Recurrence Rates* in
846 Patients
(Stages 0, I and II)

	No. Survivors/ Total No. Patients	%
Stage 0	0/116	0.0
Stage I	20/397	5.0
Stage II	46/333	13.8
Stages I and II	66/730	9.0
Stages 0, I and II	66/846	7.8
Axillary recurrences		
Stages I and II	6/730	0.8
Stages 0, I and II	6/846	0.7

*Only 2.9% of patients were skin grafted.

Table 3. Staging System:
Potentially Curable Breast Cancer

Stage 0			
In situ (Noninvasive)	TIS		
Invasive			
No evidence of tumor	T0	N0	M0
	T1ai		
Tumor up to 0.5 cm $- - - - - - - -$		N0	M0
	T1bi		
	T1aii		
Tumor 0.5 to 0.9 cm $- - - - - - -$		N0	M0
	T1bii		
Stage I (Invasive)			
	T1aiii		
Tumor 1.0 to 1.9 cm $- - - - - - -$		N0	M0
	T1biii		
	T2a		
Tumor 2.0 to 5.0 cm $- - - - - - -$		N0	M0
	T2b		
	T3a		
Tumor over 5 cm $- - - - - - -$		N0	M0
	T3b		
Stage II (Invasive)			
Positive, nonfixed homo-	T0	N1b	M0
lateral axillary nodes	T1	N1b	M0
	T2	N1b	M0
	T3	N1b	M0

Our stage 0, which we also call preclinical, presymptomatic or occult, refers to a cancer that is less than the 1-cm size that is usually needed for palpation [66] and without evidence of nodal involvement or distant metastases. It can be either noninvasive (in situ) or invasive. Stage 0 includes TIS (in situ cancers) and invasive cancers, i.e. T0 (no evidence of primary tumor), T1ai and T1bi (tumors less than 0.5 cm) and T1aii and T1bii (tumors 0.5 to 9.9 cm), all of which are N0, M0.

Stage I refers to palpable tumors without evidence of nodal involvement. It inclues T1aiii and T1biii (tumors 1.0 to 1.9 cm), T2a and T2b (tumors 2 to 5 cm) and T3a and T3b (tumors over 5 cm), all of which are N0, M0.

Stage II refers to a lesion with positive homolateral axillary nodes that are not fixed. It includes T0-, T1-, T2- and T3-sized tumors, all of which are N1b but M0. Other classifications put T3 tumors, larger than 5 cm, in the class of stage III, even though they are N0, M0 or N1b, M0.

Skin dimpling, minimal skin edema over the tumor, nipple retraction and elevation do not influence the classification. Fixation of the tumor to the underlying pectoral fascia and/or muscle does not alter the classification of potentially curable, but fixation to the chest wall places the lesion in the stage III classification.

Comparative Results with Different Approaches

Our ten-year survival and recurrence rates compare favorably with those from centers using other approaches (Table 4). The absolute ten-year survival rates and local recurrence rates for patients with potentially curable breast cancers treated by various approaches were as follows:

Table 4. Potentially Curable Breast Cancer:
Comparison of Statistics

	No. Patients	10-Year Survival	Local Recurrence
Conservative selective surgery (Crile – Cleveland Clinic [18])	453	45.0%	7.0%*
Radical selective surgery (Urban – Memorial Sloan-Kettering [32])	564	61.0%	7.7%
Moderate selective surgery (Leis – New York Medical College)	846	63.0%	7.8%†
Primary radiotherapy (Calle – Foundation Curie [44])	514	51.0%	S_1 12.0% ‡ S_2 55.0%
Adjuvant chemotherapy (NSABP – National Cancer Institute [52]) (Predominately radical mastectomies)	826	46.0%	

*Axillary recurrences are not included.
†Only 2.9% of patients were skin grafted.
‡About 33% required secondary mastectomies.

1. A survival rate of 45% and a local recurrence rate of 7%, which did not include axillary recurrences, for 453 patients treated at the Cleveland Clinic [18] by the conservative selective surgical approach.
2. A survival rate of 61% and a local recurrence rate of 7.7% for 565 patients treated at the Memorial Sloan-Kettering Cancer Center [32] by the radical selective surgical approach.
3. A survival rate of 63% and a local recurrence rate of 7.8% for 846 patients treated at the New York Medical College Affiliated Hospitals by the moderate selective surgical approach.
4. A survival rate of 51%, with a persistent or recurrent disease rate of 12%, for those patients with tumors less than 3 cm in size and without clinically involved nodes, and 55% for those with tumors larger than 3 cm with clinically involved nodes for 370 of 514 patients treated at the Foundation Curie [44] by primary radiotherapy. About 33% of the patients with persistent or recurrent disease required secondary mastectomies.
5. A survival rate of 46% for 826 patients from 23 participating institutions reported by the National Surgical Adjuvant Breast Cancer Project in 1975 [52], in which the predominant type of operation was a radical mastectomy. Limited adjuvant chemotherapy was also utilized.

The Other-Breast Results

Prophylactic removal of the other breast was performed in 112 patients who were in the high-risk group for developing cancer in it, although there were no adverse clinical or x-ray changes. There were 19 (16.9%) unsuspected cancers, of which 12 (63.2%) were noninvasive and 7 (36.8%) were invasive. Another 21 patients (18.7%) had atypias. The absolute (no evidence of disease) survival rate for 48 patients followed for ten or more years was 92.3%.

In a series of 321 random biopsies of the other breast in 500 patients undergoing definitive surgery for cancer in their first breast, 7.5% were found to have cancers; of these, 41.7% were invasive and 58.3% were noninvasive. Another 15.3% had atypias, for a combined figure of 22.7% for atypias and cancers.

The reported yield of cancers from random biopsies in other series is at considerable variance, ranging from 4.5% to 12.5% [54]. The rate of detection correlates with the diligence of the examining pathologist and the size of the biopsy. Biopsy specimens of 4 to 5 cm give the highest rates, while token biopsies have a very low yield. Another factor is whether or not clinically and mammographically suspicious areas are included [53, 54] as random biopsies. We do not include these in our group.

Cosmetic and Functional Results

Since the majority of patients in our series had less than radical mastectomies, there was an increased percentage of better arm and shoulder function and a decreased percentage of significant arm edema (which can be disabling as well as disfiguring), as compared to series with radical surgical approaches.

The overall cosmetic appearance was also better than in more radical approaches. The appearance after a modified radical mastectomy or lesser procedure is much better than after a radical mastectomy with its noticeable axillary and subclavicular hollows and prominent washboard appearance of the ribs. A carefully performed modified radical mastectomy, which was the most commonly used operation in our series, can offer a cosmetic appearance on a par with a simple mastectomy.

Finally, with the preservation of at least the pectoralis major muscle in the majority of our patients, a satisfactory breast reconstruction was possible in properly selected patients without much difficulty.

While the appearance of a patient can never be restored to that of her premastectomy state, restorative surgery offers a great deal. Our patients have been especially grateful for not having to wear an external prosthesis, for their appearance in a bra, in a tube top, in a swimming suit or in an evening dress.

Summary

The surgeon's role of primary importance in the care of the breast cancer patient is emphasized and a description of the various types of surgical procedures, with special reference to the different types of modified radical mastectomies, is presented.

The current evaluation studies by the NSABP, the criteria used for the selection of procedures, the major types of selective surgical approaches, the role of primary radiotherapy, the changing picture from radical to lesser surgical procedures, the NIH Consensus Conference recommendations and the importance of obtaining hormone receptor studies are discussed.

A moderate selective surgical approach is presented, along with a discussion about the management of the other breast and the role of restorative surgery. The results in 846 patients with potentially curable breast cancers followed for ten or more years, in which 80.3% had less than radical mastectomy, are presented — with an absolute, no evidence of disease survival rate of 63% and a local recurrence rate of 7.8%, with less than 2.9% of the patients having been skin grafted. These results are compared to those obtained with other types of surgical approaches and with primary radiotherapy.

References

1. Silverberg, E.: Cancer statistics 1979. CA 29:6, 1979.
2. Cammarata, A., Rosen, P.P. and Leis, H.P., Jr.: Breast biopsy: Surgical aspects, role of frozen section and specimen radiograpy. *In* Gallager, H.S., Leis, H.P., Jr., Snyderman, R.K. and Urban, J.A. (eds.): The Breast. St. Louis:C. V. Mosby Co., 1978.
3. Leis, H.P., Jr. and Girolamo, R.: Preoperative work-up in breast cancer. Int. Surg. J. 63:17, 1978.
4. Fisher, B.: The operative management of primary breast cancer. *In* Rubin, P. (ed.): Updated Breast Cancer. New York:American Cancer Society, Inc., 1978.
5. Fisher, B.: Breast cancer management: Alternatives to radical mastectomy. N. Engl. J. Med. 301:326, 1979.
6. Black, M.M.: Immunopathology of breast cancer. *In* Ioachim, H.L. (ed): Pathology Annual. New York:Appleton-Century-Crofts, 1977.
7. Black, M. and Zachrau, R.E.: Immunotherapy of breast cancer. *In* Gallager, H.S., Leis, H.P., Jr., Snyderman, R.K. and Urban, J.A. (eds.): The Breast. St. Louis:C. V. Mosby Co., 1978.
8. McGuire, W.L.: Estrogens and other receptors: Principles and clinical applications. *In* Gallager, H.S., Leis, H.P., Jr., Snyderman, R.K. and Urban, J.A. (eds.): The Breast. St. Louis:C. V. Mosby Co., 1978.

9. NIH Consensus Conference: Steroid receptors in Breast Cancer, vol. 2, no. 6, 1979.

10. Black, M.M. and Kwon, C.S.: Prognostic factors in breast cancer. *In* Gallager, H.S., Leis, H.P., Jr., Snyderman, R.K. and Urban, J.A. (eds.): The Breast. St. Louis:C. V. Mosby Co., 1978.

11. Fisher, E.R. and Fisher, B.: Relationship of pathologic and some clinical discriminants to the spread of breast cancer. *In* Rubin, P. (ed.): Updated Breast Cancer. New York:American Cancer Society, Inc., 1978.

12. Leis, H.P., Jr.: Criteria and standards for evaluation of treatment results. *In* Gallager, H.S., Leis, H.P., Jr., Snyderman, R.K. and Urban, J.A. (eds.): The Breast. St. Louis:C. V. Mosby Co., 1978.

13. Nealon, T.: Treatment of stage 1 carcinoma of the breast using histologic grading. Presented at ACS Science Writer's Seminar, March 1979.

14. Leis, H.P., Jr.: The Surgeon's dilemma in breast cancer. J. Breast 1:30, 1975.

15. Leis, H.P., Jr.: Selective moderate surgical approach for potentially curable breast cancer. *In* Gallager, H.S., Leis, H.P., Jr., Snyderman, R.K. and Urban, J.A. (eds.): The Breast. St. Louis:C. V. Mosby Co., 1978.

16. Leis, H.P., Jr.: Selective and reconstructive surgical procedures for carcinoma of the breast. Surg. Gynecol. Obstet. 148:17, 1979.

17. Leis, H.P., Jr.: Breast cancer surgery in the United States and Canada: Current practice. Int. Surg. 65:201, 1980.

18. Crile, G.C., Jr.: Results of conservative treatment of breast cancer at 10 and 15 years. Ann. Surg. 181:26, 1975.

19. Hermann, R.E.: Selective conservative treatment of early breast cancer. J. Breast 2:41, 1976.

20. Hermann, R.E., Esselstyn, C.B., Jr. and Crile, G.C., Jr.: Conservative surgical treatment of potentially curable breast cancer. *In* Gallager, H.S., Leis, H.P., Jr., Snyderman, R.K. and Urban, J.A. (eds.): The Breast. St. Louis:C. V. Mosby Co., 1978.

21. NIH Consensus Conference: The Treatment of Primary Breast Cancer: Management of Local Disease, vol. 2, no. 5, 1979.

22. Reynier, Jr., Mogenet, M., Santos, J.P. et al: Subcutaneous mastectomy in the treatment of cancer of the breast. Int. Surg. 63:17, 1979.

23. Auchincloss, H.: Significance of location and number of axillary metastases in carcinoma of the breast. Ann. Surg. 158:37, 1963.

24. Caceras, E., Lingan, M. and Delgado, P.: Evaluation of dissection of the axilla in modified radical mastectomy. Surg. Gynecol. Obstet. 143:395, 1976.

25. Madden, J.L.: Modified radical mastectomy. Surg. Gynecol. Obstet. 121:1221, 1965.

26. Kodama, H.: Modification of muscle-preserving radical mastectomy. Cancer 44:1517, 1979.

27. Schmitz, R.L.: The wound in modified radical mastectomy. Surg. Gynecol. Obstet. 149:738, 1979.

28. Patey, D.H. and Dyson, W.H.: The prognosis of carcinoma of the breast in relation to the type of operation performed. Br. J. Cancer 2:71, 1948.
29. Handley, R.S.: The conservative radical mastectomy of Patey: 10 year results in 427 patients. J. Dis. Breast 2:16, 1976.
30. Roses, D.F., Harris, M.N. and Gumport, S.L.: Total mastectomy with axillary gland dissection (a modified radical mastectomy). Am. J. Surg. 134:674, 1977.
31. Halsted, W.S.: The results of operations for cure of cancer of the breast performed at Johns Hopkins Hospital from June 1889 to January 1894. Johns Hopkins Med. J. 4:297, 1894-95.
32. Urban, J.A.: Selective radical surgical treatment for primary breast cancer. In Gallager, H.S., Leis, H.P., Jr., Snyderman, R.K. and Urban, J.A. (eds.): The Breast. St. Louis:C. V. Mosby Co., 1978.
33. Gallager, H.S. and Martin, J.E.: The study of mammary carcinoma by correlated mammography and subserial whole organ sectioning. Cancer 23:855, 1969.
34. Rosen, P.P., Fracchia, Urban, J.A. et al: "Residual" mammary carcinoma following simulated partial mastectomy. Cancer 35:739, 1975.
35. Schmitz, R.L.: The Breast Cancer Survey of the Commission on Cancer. American College of Surgeons, 1979, p. 17.
36. Surgeons back radical mastectomy. Med. World News, Nov. 8, 1974, p. 21.
37. Baker, R.R., Montague, A.C. and Childs, J.N.: A comparison of modified radical mastectomy to radical mastectomy in the treatment of operable breast cancer. Ann. Surg. 189:553, 1979.
38. Fox, M.S.: Diagnosis and treatment of breast cancer. JAMA 241:489, 1979.
39. Lesnick, G.: Surgical treatment of breast cancer. N.Y. State J. Med. 79:211, 1979.
40. Montoro, A.F. and Monteiro, D.M.: Comparison of axillary nodes in modified and radical mastectomy procedures. J. Brazil. Coll. Surg. 3:234, 1976.
41. Alpert, S., Ghossein, N.A., Stacey, P. et al: Primary management of operable breast cancer by minimal surgery and radiotherapy. Cancer 42:2054, 1978.
42. Atkins, H., Hayward, J.L., Klugman, D.J. et al: Treatment of early breast cancer; A report after ten years of clinical trial. Br. Med. J. 2:423, 1972.
43. Bataini, J.P., Picco, C., Martin, M. et al: Relationship between time-dose and local control of operable breast cancer treated by tumorectomy and radiotherapy or by radical radiotherapy alone. Cancer 42:2059, 1978.
44. Calle, R., Pilleron, J.P., Schlienger, P. et al: Conservative management of operable breast cancer by primary radiotherapy. Cancer 42:2045, 1978.
45. Harris, J.R. and Levene, M.B.: The role of radiation therapy in the

primary treatment of cancer of the breast. Semin. Oncol. 5:403, 1978.

46. Montague, E.: Radiotherapy as primary modality in treatment of curable breast cancer. *In* Gallager, H.S., Leis, H.P., Jr., Snyderman, R.K. and Urban, J.A. (eds.): The Breast. St. Louis:C. V. Mosby Co., 1978.
47. Pantoja, E., Frede, T. and Kunchala, S.: Complications of postoperative radiation in breast cancer. J. Breast 4:4, 1979.
48. Prosnitz, L.R., Goldenberg, I.S., Packard, R.A. et al: Radiation therapy as initial treatment for early stage cancer of the breast without mastectomy. Cancer 39:917, 1977.
49. Weber, E. and Hellman, S.: Radiation as primary treatment for local control of breast carcinoma. JAMA 234:608, 1975.
50. Wise, L., Mason, A.Y. and Ackerman, L.V.: Local excision and irradiation. Ann. Surg. 174:392, 1971.
51. Wizenberg, M.J.: Carcinoma of the breast. Surg. Gynecol. Obstet. 149:321, 1979.
52. Fisher, B., Slack, N., Katrych, D. et al: Ten year follow-up results of patients with carcinomas of the breast in a co-operative clinical trial evaluating surgical adjuvant chemotherapy. Surg. Gynecol. Obstet. 140:528, 1975.
54. Leis, H.P., Jr.: Management of the remaining breast. Cancer 46:1026, 1980.
54. Leis, H.P., Jr.: Management of the remaining breast. Cancer (In press.)
55. Leis, H.P., Jr.: Epidemiology of breast cancer: Identification of the high-risk women. *In* Gallager, H.S., Leis, H.P., Jr., Snyderman, R.K. and Urban, J.A. (eds.): The Breast. St. Louis:C. V. Mosby Co., 1978.
56. Leis, H.P., Jr. and Raciti, A.: The search for the high-risk patient for breast cancer. *In* Stoll, B.A. (ed.): Risk Factors in Breast Cancer. London:William Heinemann Medical Books Ltd., 1976.
57. Leis, H.P., Jr. and Kwon, C.S.: Fibrocystic disease of the breast. J. Reprod. Med. 22:291, 1979.
58. Wolfe, J.N.: Risk for breast cancer development determined by mammographic parenchymal pattern. Cancer 37:2486, 1976.
59. Byrne, R.: Utilization of thermography as a risk indicator in breast cancer. J. Dis. Breast 2:43, 1976.
60. Allison, A.B. and Howorth, M.B., Jr.: Carcinoma in a nipple preserved by heterotopic auto-implantation. N. Engl. J. Med. 298:1132, 1978.
61. Bouvier, B.: Problems in breast reconstruction. Med. J. Aust. 1:937, 1977.
62. Dowden, R.V., Horton, C.E., Rosato, F.E. et al: Reconstruction of the breast after mastectomy. Surg. Gynecol. Obstet. 149:109, 1979.
63. Smith, J., Payne, W.S. and Carney, J.A.: Involvement of the nipple and areola in carcinoma of the breast. Surg. Gynecol. Obstet. 143:546, 1976.
64. Snyderman, R.K.: Reconstruction of the breast. *In* Gallager, H.S., Leis, H.P., Jr., Snyderman, R.K. and Urban, J.A. (eds.): The Breast. St. Louis:C. V. Mosby Co., 1978.

65. American Joint Committee Handbook on Classification and Staging of Cancer by Site, Staging of Cancer of the Breast. Chicago:American Joint Committee, 1978, pp. 101-104.
66. Leis, H.P., Jr.: Minimal breast cancer. Mod. Med. 75:58, 1975.

Self-Evaluation Quiz

1. In 1979, in the United States alone, there were about _____ new cases of breast cancer.
   a) 66,000
   b) 76,000
   c) 86,000
   d) 96,000
   e) 106,000
2. As related to the surgeon's role in the treatment of breast cancer all of the following are true *except*:
   a) He removes the tumor load rapidly
   b) He does not disturb immunocompetence
   c) He provides for pathological staging by removing the axillary lymph nodes
   d) He offers the patient a good systemic control of her cancer
   e) He supplies tissue for study of the growth potential or virulence of the cancer
3. In a conservative or limited modified radical mastectomy which one of the following is true?
   a) All levels of axillary nodes are removed
   b) Rotter's nodes are removed
   c) Both pectoral muscles are preserved
   d) The internal mammary nodes are sampled
   e) A latissimus dorsi myocutaneous flap is used
4. In the 1971 NSABP protocol women were randomized into three therapy groups: radical mastectomy, total mastectomy and total mastectomy with regional radiotherapy.
   a) True
   b) False
5. All patients in the three groups of the 1976 NSABP protocol who had positive axillary nodes received adjuvant chemotherapy.
   a) True
   b) False

6. In the criteria for selective surgery as related to tumor growth potential or virulence, all of the following are used *except*:
   a) The histologic type of the tumor
   b) Whether the tumor is invasive or not
   c) The stage, size and location of the cancer
   d) Whether there is central tumor necrosis or not
   e) The growth pattern of the tumor
7. The three main types of selective surgical approaches for patients with potentially curable breast cancers are conservative, moderate and radical.
   a) True
   b) False
8. Today the most popular procedure in the United States for patients with potentially curable breast cancers is:
   a) Simple mastectomy
   b) Partial mastectomy
   c) Modified radical mastectomy
   d) Radical mastectomy
   e) Extended radical mastectomy
9. The NIH Consensus Conference in 1979 on "The Treatment of Primary Breast Cancer: Management of Local Disease" recommended that a procedure that preserves the pectoral muscles, i.e. a total mastectomy with axillary dissection, should be recognized as the current treatment standard for women who have stage I and selected stage II breast cancers.
   a) True
   b) False
10. Even in preclinical invasive cancers less than 1 cm in size, axillary dissection of the first level of nodes should be done since metastases do occur.
    a) True
    b) FaLse
11. Patients at high risk for developing cancer in their other breast include all of the following *except*:
    a) Those with early, good prognostic cancers
    b) Those with multicentric cancers in the first breast
    c) Those with scirrhous carcinomas in the first breast
    d) Those with a family history of breast cancer
    e) Those with an abnormal thermogram in the remaining breast

12. The reported results with the moderate selective surgical
    approach are on a par with, or better than, the conservative
    and radical selective surgical approaches, primary radio-
    therapy and the 1975 NSABP report in which the pre-
    dominant type of operation was the radical mastectomy.
    a) True
    b) False

13. The rate of detection of cancers by random biopsies of the
    other breast correlates with the diligence of the examining
    pathologist and the size of the biopsy.
    a) True
    b) False

14. In view of the possibility of doing restorative surgery,
    efforts should be made, if it does not jepordize the patient's
    chance for cure, to do all of the following *except*:
    a) Make transverse or oblique incisions
    b) Preserve the pectoralis major muscle
    c) Avoid skin grafting
    d) Avoid removing the fascia over the pectoralis major
       muscle
    e) Avoid kilovoltage radiotherapy to the chest wall

Answers on page 335.

Treatment Considerations in In Situ Breast Cancer

Sven J. Kister, M.D.

Objective

The purpose of this paper is to present the choices of management and treatment of two so-called in situ breast carcinomas and the relevant data in support of each.

Two pathologic entities probably comprise what are commonly termed "in situ carcinomas" of the breast: namely intraductal carcinoma and in situ lobular carcinoma. At Columbia we call in situ intraductal carcinoma, intraductal carcinoma and lobular carcinoma in situ, lobular neoplasia.

Although both lesions are easily diagnosed by most pathologists, they are hard to define in terms of their behavior. This presentation is a brief review of the data available from the literature and from our institutional experience. The discussion will at times be oversimplified and editorialized, reflecting to some degree the uncertainties of knowledge about these lesions.

Intraductal Carcinoma in Which Invasion Is Not Demonstrated (IDC-IND)

I prefer the term "IDC-IND" to "in situ intraductal carcinoma" or to simply "intraductal carcinoma" because it is more precise in defining the state of our present histologic capabilities. IDC-IND is a true carcinoma. The individual cells of this lesion are histologically malignant. By light microscopy the cells are confined to the ducts only and do not invade the

Sven J. Kister, M.D., Associate Clinical Professor of Surgery, Columbia University, College of Physicians and Surgeons, New York, N.Y.

surrounding stroma. Individual cells of IDC-IND are usually indistinguishable from individual cells of invasive intraductal carcinoma. These lesions are rarely found clinically. Most are diagnosed by mammography, where they appear as microcalcifications, or incidentally in biopsy sections which were taken for another clinically detectable lesion.

Since our surgical pathology department recognizes only intraductal or intraductal invasive carcinoma, we have no individual or institutional data about IDC-IND. I have, instead, summarized the data available from the literature and they are as presented in Table 1.

The total number of cases from the three studies reviewed is only 132 [1-3]. These represent patients who underwent mastectomy following the diagnosis of IDC-IND on previous biopsy. Residual IDC-IND was present in 58% and invasive IDC in 14% of mastectomy specimens. In 33% of specimens no residual carcinoma was found. Furthermore, residual carcinoma in the mastectomy specimens outside the biopsy quadrant was found by Rosen et al in 33% of patients [1]. Progression to ipsilateral invasive IDC occurred in 40% of patients not treated by mastectomy in the study reported by Betsill et al [4]. Axillary lymph node metastases were reported by Carter and Smith in 4 of 29 cases, in 1 case when the primary lesion was IDC-IND and in 3 when the primary lesion was invasive IDC. Risk of developing an IDC-IND in the opposite breast is estimated to be equal to the higher risk associated with all second primary carcinomas of the contralateral breast.

Table 1. Intraductal Carcinoma — Invasion Not Demonstrated: Residual Carcinoma in Mastectomy Specimen After Excisional Biopsy for IDC-IND

Source	Residual Carcinoma in Breast	
	Noninvasive	Invasive
Rosen et al, 1979 [1] 53 cases	64%	6%
Carter and Smith, 1977 [2] 38 cases	66%	18%
Shah et al, 1973 [3] 45 cases	47%	18%

At Columbia we consider all intraductal carcinomas as potentially invasive and capable of metastasizing.

Treatment of IDC-IND should be based on the above-mentioned data because IDC-IND cells are identical to IDC invasive cells. IDC-IND is multicentric, and progression from IDC-IND to invasive IDC seems to occur in almost half of the patients. Therefore a total mastectomy is the preferred method of treatment. An axillary dissection should follow. Although axillary metastases are infrequent, knowledge of axillary lymph node status is important in deciding the need for adjuvant treatment. The uninvolved opposite breast should be followed closely with physical examinations at four-month intervals and mammograms at about yearly intervals, particularly when the patient is postmenopausal.

Lobular Neoplasia (LN) or Lobular Carcinoma In Situ

In contrast to IDC-IND, lobular neoplasia is probably not a true carcinoma. The individual cells are histologically not malignant. They are regular in size and shape. Their nuclei are uniform and rarely seen in mitosis. These cells are distinctly different from mammary carcinoma cells. LN cells are confined to the lobules and terminal ducts. LN does not metastasize. LN and true infiltrating carcinoma may be present simultaneously in the same biopsy specimen. If this is the case, the diagnosis is, of course, carcinoma in association with LN. It should be recognized and treated as such. This discussion is limited to lobular neoplasia occurring alone, without simultaneous carcinoma. Several reports of this benign lobular proliferation have been recently published, most notably the studies by Haagensen et al [5] and Rosen et al [6]. A summary of these studies is presented in Table 2. It is evident from these studies that LN is not a clinical entity, because it does not produce a palpable mass, is not detectable by mammography (if mammograms show some findings, they are associated with an adjacent and usually benign lesion), and is always an incidental finding detected by the pathologist studying tissues from a biopsy usually performed for a benign breast disease, most commonly cysts. Its true incidence in the general female population is

VANDERBILT MEDICAL CENTER LIBRARY

Table 2. Lobular Neoplasia

	Haagensen et al [5], Columbia-Presbyterian, 1977	Rosen et al [6], Memorial Hospital, 1978	Kister, Columbia-Presbyterian, 1980
Years covered by study	1930-1972		1972-1980
Commonest age of occurrence	40-50 Years	40-49 Years	40-50 Years
Range of age	25-80 Years	28-78 Years	37-69 Years
% Premenopausal	90%	70%	70%
No. of patients	211	99	40
Commonest lesion for which biopsy done	Cysts	Cysts	Cysts
Length of follow-up in years			
Range	1-42 Years	–	1-18 Years
Mean	14 Years	24 Years	5 Years
Interval between diagnosis of LN and occurrence of carcinoma			
1-10 Years	63%	30%	100%
11-25 Years	32%	60%	
>25 Years	5%	10%	
Subsequent carcinoma			
No. of patients	36 (17%)	32 (32%)	4 (10%)
Side	Ipsi = Contra	Ipsi = Contra	Ipsi = Contra
Incidence (× normal)	7	9	
Small-cell type	33%	40%	0
Greatest cumulative probability of developing carcinoma in 25 years	25%	–	–
Follow-up status unknown	1/211	15/99	0
Number of patients dying of breast cancer	6	9	0

therefore not known. LN is mostly found in premenopausal women, at least in its lobular component, and regresses with menopause. The ductal phase is most commonly present in postmenopausal women. LN is multicentric, multilobular and bilateral in a high percentage of patients. About 25% of women with LN will develop a true carcinoma in their lifetime. The carcinomas that develop in these women are small-cell type in one third of the cases. The rest of the carcinomas vary in histologic type, belonging mostly to those varieties associated with a better prognosis, e.g. tubular, intraductal, solid circumscribed and apocrine. The carcinomas develop with equal likelihood in either breast. No histologic characteristics have proved to be helpful in predicting which patients are more likely to develop a true carcinoma. LN is a relatively rare lesion. The greatest majority of women with carcinoma of the breast show no histologic evidence of previous or simultaneous LN.

In Haagensen's series of 211 women, six died of carcinoma of the breast. In all six the diagnosis of LN was missed in the original biopsy specimen. These women, therefore, were not recognized as high-risk patients and were not subject to planned follow-up. In my own series of 40 women with LN, almost all were diagnosed after 1972. My data fit well into the overall pattern of the other studies. Since my series was collected prospectively and the patients followed optimally, no patients have died from breast cancer in this relatively short follow-up period.

From a host of contributing factors discussed above, the following bear directly on the management and treatment of LN: First, LN is not a clinical entity since it has no clinical symptoms or signs. Second, carcinoma following LN occurs in either the ipsilateral or contralateral breast with equal frequency. Third, there are no known histologic features predicting or identifying which patients will develop carcinoma. Only two forms of treatment seem possible and reasonable from the data, either observation or prophylactic bilateral total mastectomies. In favor of the choice of observation are the long intervals between diagnosis of LN and development of subsequent carcinoma (in 50% to 60%, over ten years), and the fact that the subsequent carcinoma is of favorable histologic type. In addition, in patients who develop a carcinoma, metastases to axillary lymph nodes are rare. No deaths have occurred during follow-up in our Columbia series. Most important, unnecessary prophylactic bilateral mastectomies in a large number of women (75%) are avoided.

In favor of the choice of bilateral mastectomy are these factors: (1) The patient is assured that carcinoma will not develop. (2) Reconstruction of both breasts is possible. (3) No anxiety produced by follow-up occurs. (4) Close and lifelong follow-up is unnecessary.

The most important factor in the management decision of LN is the patient herself. She must be completely aware of all the risks of lobular neoplasia. She must also know that our present knowledge of LN is incomplete and, therefore, still controversial.

As for my own patients, I presented all of them with information which is contained in a brief paper entitled "About Lobular Neoplasia." None of the 40 women chose bilateral mastectomies. The following case report serves well to illustrate management of in situ carcinomas.

A 47-year-old woman consulted me because of spontaneous nipple discharge from the right breast. Historically, her mother had had breast cancer premenopausally and she herself had had several cysts aspirated from both breasts. Physical examination of her breasts showed a pressure point at the 10 o'clock axis at the areolar margin of the right breast. The left breast contained a mass. Attempted aspiration of this mass failed to yield fluid. Bilateral biopsies were recommended and were performed. At the right breast exploration, a single dilated duct was identified and excised with only minimal normal tissue about the duct. Upon opening the duct in the operating room, a typical intraductal papilloma was seen. The left breast exploration showed gross cystic disease. No frozen sections were done. Paraffin sections 24 hours later confirmed the diagnoses of intraductal papilloma and gross cystic disease. In addition, bilateral LN was present. The patient was given the usual information about LN. She chose observation per our recommendation. In April 1976 she had a negative breast examination and mammography which showed microcalcifications in the right breast. In

June 1976, the calcifications were excised with specimen mammography control. Intraductal carcinoma and LN were found. A total mastectomy and axillary dissection were recommended and performed at the end of June 1976. The mastectomy specimen showed no residual IDC but showed LN. All 25 axillary lymph nodes were negative for metastases. Follow-up continued. In March 1977, a cyst in the left breast was again aspirated. In November 1979 physical examination was negative. Mammograms at that visit showed microcalcifications in the left breast. Excision of calcifications from the left breast showed an intraductal carcinoma, possibly intraductal invasive carcinoma. A left total mastectomy with axillary lymph node dissection was performed. The mastectomy specimen showed residual intraductal carcinoma and intraductal invasive carcinoma. All 36 lymph nodes were free of metastases. To date she is well.

It seems obvious from the data that our present knowledge about these two in situ carcinomas, particularly LN, is insufficient to categorically recommend what is probably prophylactic surgery. Yet, in most institutions in our country, a patient with LN will be advised to have an ipsilateral modified radical mastectomy or bilateral simple mastectomies. It is also obvious that histologic methodology has been exhausted to identify biologic behavior of these in situ carcinomas. What we need are finer, more sophisticated probes, possibly of the immunobiochemical variety, to predict the biologic behavior of LN.

References

1. Rosen, P.P., Senie, R., Schottenfeld, D. and Ashikari, R.: Noninvasive breast carcinoma. Ann. Surg. 189:377-382, 1979.
2. Carter, D. and Smith, R.R.L.: Carcinoma in situ of the breast. Cancer 40:1189-1193, 1977.
3. Shah, J.P., Rosen, P.P. and Robbins, G.F.: Pitfalls of local excision in the treatment of carcinoma of the breast. Surg. Gynecol. Obstet. 136:721-725, 1973.
4. Betsill, W., Rosen, P.P., Lieberman, P.H. and Robbins, G.F.: Intraductal carcinoma: Long-term follow-up after treatment by biopsy alone. JAMA 239:1863-1867, 1978.

5. Haagensen, C.D., Lane, N. and Lattes, R.: Lobular neoplasia (so-called lobular carcinoma in situ) of the breast. Cancer 42:737-769, 1978.
6. Rosen, P.P., Lieberman, P.H., Braun, D.W., Jr. et al: Lobular carcinoma in situ of the breast. Am. J. Surg. Pathol. 2:225, 1978.

Self-Evaluation Quiz

1. Two "in situ" breast cancers are intraductal carcinoma and lobular neoplasia.
   a) True
   b) False
2. IDC-IND is not a true carcinoma.
   a) True
   b) False
3. IDC-IND is not detectable by mammography.
   a) True
   b) False
4. The surgical treatment of IDC-IND should at least include a mastectomy.
   a) True
   b) False
5. LN is not a true cancer.
   a) True
   b) False
6. LN is not detectable by mammography.
   a) True
   b) False
7. LN is sometimes associated with a true cancer. Treatment of such a lesion should be:
   a) Ipsilateral subcutaneous mastectomy
   b) Bilateral total mastectomies
   c) Observation with close follow-up
   d) Total mastectomy with axillary dissection of the ipsilateral breast
   e) Adjuvant chemotherapy
8. LN is not multricentric and rarely if ever occurs in the opposite breast.
   a) True
   b) False

9. Both IDC-IND and LN are relatively rare lesions.
   a) True
   b) False
10. IDC-IND is multicentric in the ipsilateral breast.
   a) True
   b) False

Answers on page 335.

Radical Mastectomy in the Treatment of Operable Breast Cancer

Charles Fineberg, M.D.

Objectives

The gradual unselective utilizing of lesser than radical mastectomy for operable breast carcinoma has reached such proportions as to jeopardize the proper treatment of the majority of patients who seek surgical help with the diagnosis of breast cancer. It is estimated that 1500 to 1800 patients are being subjected to death each year because of inadequate surgery. The objective of this presentation is to present definitive evidence which shows that patients are being subjected to lesser than radical mastectomy without any knowledge of the size of the lesion involved, the type of malignancy involved or the extent of regional node involvement. Evidence is also presented showing that even in the most favorable cases, the so-called minimal carcinomas, a significant number of patients already have extensive lymph node involvement.

The supposition that all axillary lymph nodes can be removed by modified mastectomy is questioned. The use of five-year statistics for any operative procedure on the breast is questioned since most patients who have breast carcinoma in which nothing is done will survive five years. A request for a more accurate and honest titling of surgical procedures is made since present titles such as total mastectomy and modified radical mastectomy are misleading and most times erroneous.

Charles Fineberg, M.D., Professor of Surgery, Jefferson Medical College, Thomas Jefferson University, Philadelphia, Pa.

215

It was the age of wisdom. It was the age of foolishness. It was the epic of belief. It was the epic of incredulity. It was the season of light. It was the season of darkness. It was the spring of hope. It was the winter of despair. We had everything before us. We had nothing before us. Some of its noisiest authorities insisted upon being received in heaven for good or evil in a superlative degree of compassion only.

These words are taken from the pen of Charles Dickens in his work, *A Tale of Two Cities*. They most succinctly describe the confused state both clinicians and patients must deal with in the treatment of breast carcinoma.

Until 40 years ago, cancer of the breast appeared to pose very few difficulties for the clinician. What other malignant neoplasm so superficially placed in an external appendage — which we understand undergoes a very orderly change from microscopic evaluation to a clinically palpable mass before extension into the axillary lymph nodes and possibly the blood stream — offers, if treated correctly, an adequate means of eradication by surgery? In what way does cancer of the breast differ from cancers of other organs, which predominantly spread by lymphatic channels? There are relatively few cancers that are not treated surgically by en bloc dissection whenever possible for their complete eradication and possible cure. Why, then, has radical mastectomy as an acceptable procedure since the turn of the century engendered such controversy and even vilification?

As a practitioner who has been interested in this subject both in the research laboratory and in my clinical practice for 29 years, I am somewhat dismayed and saddened by the ever-increasing acceptance by surgeons in the United States of lesser and varied methods for the treatment of primary invasive breast carcinoma. This disturbing trend, which Dr. C. D. Haagensen most recently and accurately described as the "great step backwards," has been reinforced by several statistical analyses, in this country and abroad, of individuals treated with lesser operations than radical mastectomy.

Of even greater significance is the fact that the physicians who champion these methods of therapy have publicized widely in the lay literature — e.g. *Ladies' Home Journal, Reader's*

Digest, Family Circle — so that the great proportion of our population, especially women, who are primarily interested in this disease, have been unfairly and erroneously influenced as to the proper method of therapy. This trend has reached such great proportions that it has become impossible to see a patient in consultation without having the patient insist upon a method of therapy other than what the attending surgeon thinks appropriate for the lesion that he has diagnosed.

It is disappointing that no one in our profession has come forward to try to combat this onslaught of powerful propaganda and, I think, questionable statistics in a similar manner by publication of this information in lay language, in the lay press, so that the public would better understand the problem instead of forming a completely one-sided, biased opinion.

It is generally considered that William Halsted and Willie Meyer originated what is properly called radical mastectomy in 1891, but other surgeons, including Moore [1] of Middlesex in London and Banks [2] in Liverpool in 1882, had already suggested the possibility of the removal of the pectoralis muscles and exploration of the axilla for carcinoma of the breast. In 1880, Samuel W. Gross [3] — professor of surgery and the father of our department here at Thomas Jefferson University Hospital — recommended the excision of the axillary contents, nodes and pectoralis major and minor muscles for the treatment of tumors in the mammary gland. This was 11 years before Halsted popularized the first so-called radical mastectomy.

The conflict of radical mastectomy over lesser surgical procedures, with or without radiation therapy, is subject to erroneous statistical interpretations. These are traceable to the presence of unrecognized bias in case selection. The criteria that have been used for diagnosis by clinical staging or any other classification or for the assignment to a particular group may arise in the criteria for selection and then be falsely attributed to factors such as the method of treatment. The usual clinical data and the possibilities of selective concentration are almost limitless. I think most statisticians looking into this complex area will support that contention.

It is not the purpose of this presentation to delve once again into the statistical quagmire which supports various surgical procedures for the treatment of breast cancer. The combined stage I and II ten-year survival rates with radical mastectomy have been adequately reported by such authors as C. D. Haagensen, Anglem, Leber, Finney, Paine and Robbins. Unfortunately, the surgical literature contains many meaningless reports based upon small or selected examples variously classified and submitted to diverse and almost unfathomable statistical manipulation. The most challenging question that the clinical surgeon must answer today is how best to treat a patient with a disease that until now has been regarded as *potentially* curable. What do we mean by a potentially curable carcinoma of the breast? I believe it means that a tumor in the breast without palpable axillary nodes or with nodes of moderate size. This group of patients would be classified in the Manchester system as stage I or II, or in the Columbia system in category A or B.

In regard to clinical staging, one must accept the fact that an extremely high rate of clinical observation error is present before operation. This error is also present postoperatively in the histological examination of lymph nodes and, especially, of the underlying muscle tissue. The latter is an important factor and one to which we have paid very little attention up until now. Pathologists experience well-known difficulty in clearing the axilla and identifying those nodes that are involved. Indeed, it is interesting that we surgeons claim to remove so many nodes and to identify so many nodes; yet the specimen can remain on the pathologist's workbench for a week and he still cannot identify the number of nodes present. Obviously, a good deal of confusion arises when one attempts comparison between series on the basis of staging, since presumably the definition of operability must differ in various centers and would be of no value unless one accepted all comers and there were no selection of patients.

The proponents of lesser than radical mastectomy probably correctly point out the rationale for lesser procedures for what has been termed "minimal carcinoma." The generally accepted view of minimal carcinoma refers to a cancer in those patients in whom the results of clinical appraisal and appropriate study limit the disease to the breast. The clinical substages of breast cancer that would be included are lobular or intraductal

Table 1. Incidence of Multicentric Foci in Minimal Cancers

Author	No. of Patients	% Multicentric Foci
Qualhein and Gall [4]	157	54
Stewart (Forrest) [5]	50	38
Morganstern et al [6]	500	31
Gallagher and Martin [7]	200	40

carcinoma in situ, noninvasive or microinvasive cancer, nonpalpable cancer and occult cancer. These would be listed in the systems of classification as T1, T2, M0, N0, Manchester stage I and Columbia category A.

The use of local excision, lumpectomy or tylectomy — or however one chooses to classify it, in what I call "verbal garbage" — for the treatment of this group of favorable patients should be discouraged. The fact that there is a very high percentage of multicentricity (Table 1) [4-7], even in these minimal carcinomas, provides powerful evidence against such local or segmental operations.

Table 2 [8-11] points out the absence of axillary metastases in certain patients with minimal carcinoma, which would make them ideal candidates for simple mastectomy, not local excision. This is the group of patients which has an excellent prognosis and long-term survival. These facts are taken out of context most of the time, especially by lay individuals and lay journals, and are used to influence patients especially for lesser surgical procedures. It should also be remembered that these

Table 2. Incidence of Axillary Lymph Node Involvement
in Minimal Cancers

Author	Type	% Axillary Node Involvement
Berger et al [8]	Microinvasive tumors 0.3 to 0.5 mm	0
Millis and Thynne [9]	In situ intraductal	0
Moskowitz et al [10]	22 = In situ 9 = Invasive <0.5 cm	0
Westbrook and Gallagher [11]	Noninvasive intraductal	1.5

C. FINEBERG

Table 3. Incidence of Positive Axillary Lymph Nodes in
Breast Cancer Cases Discovered by Mammography Alone

Author	No. of Patients	% Positive Axillary Nodes
Barker et al [12]	13	25
Frankl and Rosenfeld [13]	75	27
Malone et al [14]	55	33
Strax [15]	54	35

extremely favorable cancers constitute a small fraction of the total incidence of breast cancers. In discussing this group of patients, it is important to emphasize the frequency of error in clinical appraisal of the extent of their disease.

The next two tables show data concerning patients with occult cancer discovered by mammography alone, and by mammography and physical examination in detection centers. Of course, individuals undergoing this type of screening would provide the most favorable group of patients for early discovery. Table 3 [12-15] shows the incidence of axillary lymph node involvement in breast cancers found originally by mammography alone. Even in this group of patients with the earliest cancers that we can possibly see, there are variations from 25% to 35% for positive axillary nodes. Table 4 [8, 10, 15-18] portrays the detection of very early carcinomas by both mammography and physical examination in detection centers. Even these patients show a high incidence of positive nodes. This is extremely important because the average incidence of nodal involvement in stage I or category A patients encountered in the ordinary practice is reported to be about 30%. Even

Table 4. Incidence of Positive Axillary Lymph Nodes in
Cancer Discovered in Detection Centers by
Mammography and Physical Examination

Author	No. of Patients	% Positive Nodes
Moskowitz et al [10]	67	24
Dowdy et al [16]	46	27
Berger et al [8]	110	30
Shapiro et al [17]	381	30
Byrd [18]	1620	23

though these are the earliest patients we are going to get, they do have significant nodal involvement.

Pickren [19] and Saphir and Amromin [20] have reported that when the axillary contents of 70% of their patients, who were supposedly free of metastasis, were subjected to a more diligent search by specific clearing methods and subserial section, an additional 33% were found to harbor metastatic disease. To use round figures, 40% to 45% of localized cancers will have involvement of the axillary nodes. This becomes a serious responsibility for the surgeon who elects to do an operative procedure that deliberately leaves behind easily removable disease, which certainly cannot be stated to be profitable for the patient.

However, the real problem surgeons face today concerns the group of patients who have invasive carcinoma of the breast. I do not wish to leave the impression that many fine surgeons in this country who do selective, careful analysis of their patients are serving them in the wrong way. I am concerned about the inappropriate treatment of individuals with invasive carcinoma in which there is no true evaluation of their pathology, and the surgeon performs less than a radical procedure without any knowledge of the detailed histology of the lesion. This change in type of surgery may be directly attributed to the patient's own misconception, or to the decision of the individual surgeon as influenced by what I believe is biased and incomplete anatomical, physiological and statistical evidence. The use of five- and six-year survival rates should be unacceptable to the surgeon as a basis for surgical treatment. It is indeed unfortunate that surgeons citing five-year survival figures and patients relying upon information based on five-year survival taken out of context would use this material as the basis for decision making. The widely publicized statistics of the Adjuvant Study on Breast Cancer, utilizing figures between four and six years postoperatively, have unduly influenced many surgeons and patients as to what may be deemed the proper method of therapy. Fifty percent of the surgeons who treat breast carcinoma do not have board certification and are readily influenced by statistics and by what they read in the journals.

Statistics on the treatment of minimal carcinoma should not be used across the board as a basis for treatment for all patients with invasive breast cancer. Proponents of radical mastectomy for the treatment of breast cancer have been accused of showing emotionalism for their failure to adopt what is termed "newer methods" and what are actually lesser operative procedures for the treatment of invasive breast carcinoma. The use of the term "emotionalism" presents an enigma since it is the opponents of radical mastectomy who have continually and publicly emphasized the anatomical handicaps of surgery of the breast. Such terminology as mutilation, deformity, horrible swelling of the arm and hollow of the chest wall has been utilized to influence the potential patient about the horrors of radical mastectomy. These descriptions, along with a highly prejudiced titling of the surgical procedures performed, create a definite bias as far as the patient's decision concerning the operative procedure she will accept.

I do not understand the multiple terms that are used for surgical procedures. The term "total mastectomy," which in general usage, I believe erroneously, describes an operation that removes just the soft tissue of the breast, is certainly much more acceptable to a patient than the term "radical mastectomy." The former label leads the patient to believe that something complete and total is being performed, while the latter leads the patient to believe a markedly disfiguring and life-threatening procedure will be undertaken. We do not use the word "radical" in the description of standard cancer operations for the alimentary tract or other areas of the body which encompass the removal of primary and lymphatic drainage of the area of the tumor. Furthermore, the term "modified radical mastectomy" is open to a great deal of interpretation, with various modifications being utilized, including division of the muscles, removal of the pectoralis minor muscle in one procedure and preservation of all muscles in another procedure. Standardization of terminology and a more honest description of the procedures being utilized, with changes in title, would be helpful to both the physician and the patient who is faced with breast cancer.

Proponents of lesser operations who utilize esthetics as part of their argument against radical mastectomy do their patients a disservice. There is no doubt that the removal of the pectoralis muscles from the chest wall leaves an anatomic deficit.

However, the overexaggerated descriptions of these deformities are certainly without basis. Several years ago, one of the leading proponents of lesser operations participated in a symposium in which I was also a participant. This surgeon, who has publicized widely the use of lesser procedures, was adamant about the esthetic effects of radical mastectomy. Yet when I presented my series of patients, 11 of whom had a radical mastectomy performed on one side and a simple mastectomy on the other, he was unable to identify the radical mastectomy in 7 of the 11 patients with their arms at their sides. When their arms were elevated, it became apparent that the pectoralis muscles had been removed, as illustrated below. The majority of these patients had lobular carcinoma, invasive on one side and in situ on the other side.

Figure 1 shows a patient 16 years after mastectomy. She had a radical mastectomy on one side and a simple mastectomy on the other side, but the difference is not noticeable with the arms down (Fig. 1A). When the arms are raised (Fig. 1B), one can identify the difference between the radical and the simple mastectomy.

Even in patients with large breasts, the deformity is not of the degree described by most advocates of simple procedures. Figure 2A shows a patient with large breasts who had a radical mastectomy. Certainly, there is an anatomic defect, but it is not the horrible situation that is usually described. With her prosthesis in place, her appearance is certainly quite acceptable (Fig. 2B).

With the ever-increasing employment of modified radical mastectomy for operable breast cancer in wider ranges, attention should be turned to several anatomic facts which have never been fully discussed. The lymphatic drainage of the breast is fairly constant. Even proponents of modified procedures will readily admit the direct piercing of both the pectoralis major and minor muscles by lymphatic channels on their way either to the internal mammary chain or to the axillary lymphatic network. Hultborn's very scientific radioactive gold injection studies of the lymphatics of the breast readily support this anatomic fact [21]. His study conclusively showed that the lymphatic drainage of the breast pierces the pectoralis muscles and extends extensively through the deep pectoral fascia plane

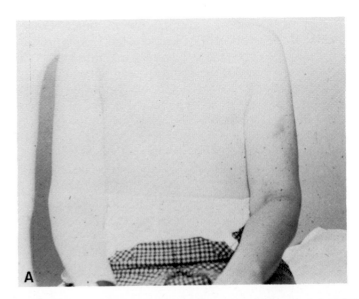

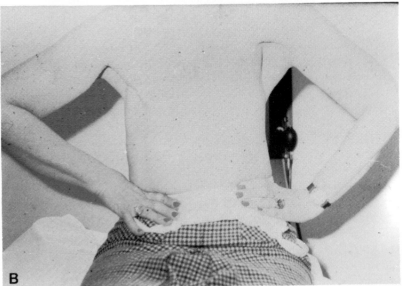

FIG. 1. Patient following radical mastectomy on one side and simple mastectomy on the other. (A) Little esthetic difference in results with arms down. (B) Difference apparent with arms raised.

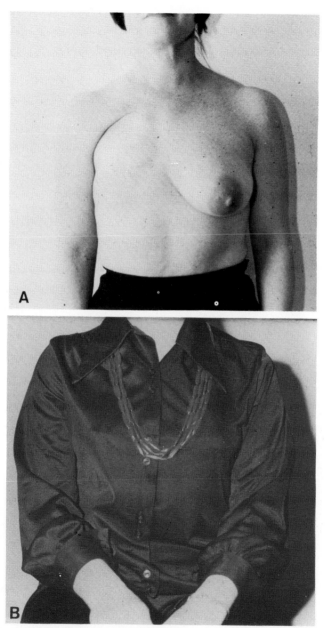

FIG. 2. Patient with large breasts, following radical mastectomy. (A) Anatomic defect. (B) Appearance with prosthesis in place.

into the lymph nodes of the dorsal surface of the pectoralis muscles (Fig. 3). The drawings of cadaver specimens readily demonstrate, although many anatomical slides do not, the direct piercing of both the pectoralis major and minor muscles by lymphatics (Fig. 4).

The variations of the modified radical mastectomy are numerous. Recent studies by Caceres [22] in Peru show a significant increase in the number of Rotter's nodes removed after modified radical mastectomy is said to have been completed. In many of the surgical techniques in which modified radical mastectomy is done, Rotter's nodes are not removed. Haagensen, in a recent review of his own histologic sections, indicated that these nodes were positive in 19% of his cases. Caceres reported that these nodes were present in 56.9% of the cases of radical mastectomies reviewed and were positive for metastasis in 17.1%. Caceres analyzed data from 50 consecutive unselected women with a mean age of 47 years. Clinical staging placed 2 patients in stage I, 43 patients in stage

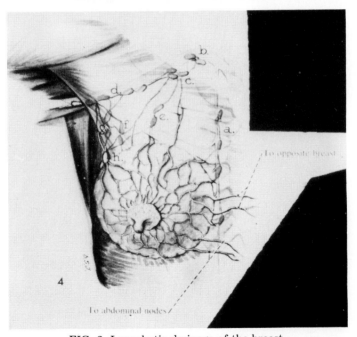

FIG. 3. Lymphatic drainage of the breast.

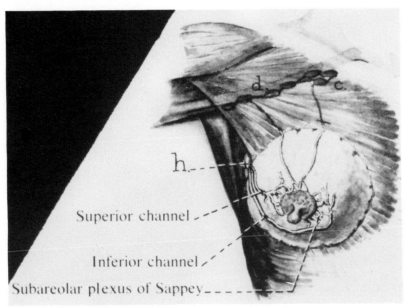

FIG. 4. Direct piercing of pectoralis major and minor muscles by lymphatics.

II, and 5 patients in stage III. The preponderance were in stage II, the usual infiltrating duct carcinoma or invasive carcinoma. Radical mastectomy was performed in two stages. The first was a modified radical mastectomy and this was completed as a radical mastectomy. Additional lymph nodes were recovered in 36 patients, with metastasis in 7. The results show that modified radical mastectomy is ineffective in eradicating lymph nodes at levels 2 and 3, and very ineffective in recovering Rotter's nodes.

In my own questioning of the various departments of pathology in Philadelphia, I have determined that adequate serial section of muscle in radical mastectomies is not uniformly or routinely performed. It therefore becomes impossible to evaluate the extent of direct lymphatic involvement in pectoral muscles underlying the breast. The fact that it occurs is readily acknowledged by some pathologists. For example, Figure 5 shows a tumor directly in the lymphatics of the pectoralis muscles, and in Figure 6 is a tumor invading the walls of the lymphatic vessels.

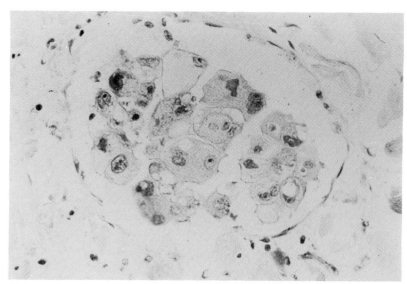

FIG. 5. Direct tumor involvement in the lymphatics of the pectoralis muscles.

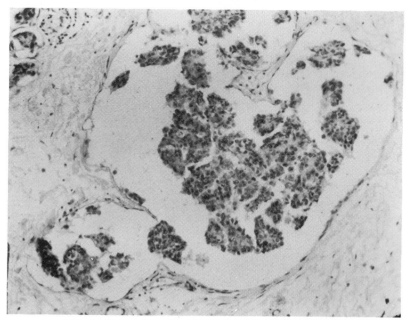

FIG. 6. Tumor invading the walls of lymphatic vessels.

There are some very interesting studies related to the pectoral muscle which are not well publicized or well known. In 1931, Wainwright [23] reported on full-section histology, in which he sectioned the entire breast of his patients and found involvement of the pectoral fascia or the pectoral muscle in 160 cases (Figs. 7 and 8). It is of interest anatomically, and most surgeons will verify the fact, that it is impossible to take all of the pectoral fascia in any type of operation except a radical mastectomy. The fascia dips down into the interstices of the pectoralis muscle. Most surgeons will admit, I think, that they pass within millimeters of the deep surface of cancer; even in intermediately located breast cancers, the surgeon passes very close and sometimes through microscopic extensions of the cancer which he can neither feel nor see.

Figure 9 shows a representative cancer from a simple mastectomy at our institution in which it is apparent that the deep fascia is involved with tumor, and the tumor has been left behind in these procedures. If it was a microscopic involvement, it is almost certain that this resection was not curative. In Figure 10 is shown a cancer from a modified radical mastectomy, with India ink used to delineate the levels of the muscle and pectoralis fascia and tumor below these levels. I defy any surgeon to tell just where the microscopic extension of cancer stops or is still present in doing this sort of token operation.

When comparing the operation which is termed radical mastectomy with lesser procedures and indicating that the results are the same, one must be aware of two invasions of truth. First, radical mastectomy which is poorly performed is worse than no operation at all. In perusing the operating room records of 350 cases at Thomas Jefferson University Hospital for the years 1935 to 1960, I found to my amazement and horror that numerous operations were performed in less than one hour. The longest length of time spent was 4½ hours, the average time was two hours, and some operations were performed in 30 minutes. It is obvious that these figures do not involve radical mastectomies. If this occurs in a teaching institution with such a solid reputation, surely there are many other institutions in which comparisons of radical and simple mastectomies and lesser procedures have been performed with this fallacy included.

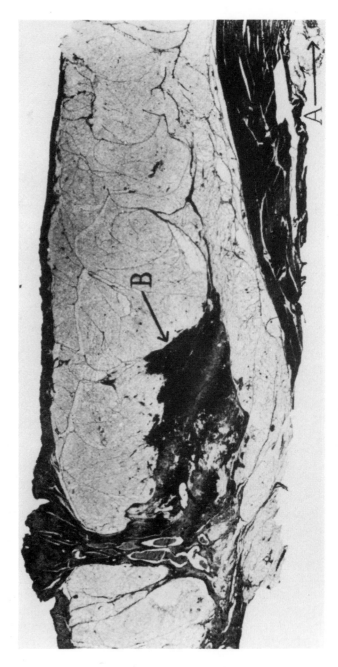

FIG. 7. Full-section view of specimen showing primary tumors at *B* and carcinoma in the pectoral muscle at *A*. (Reprinted from Wainwright [23]. By permission of Surgery, Gynecology & Obstetrics.)

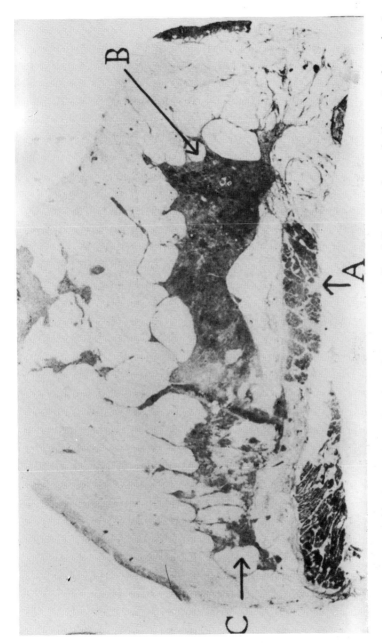

FIG. 8. Full-section view of specimen showing primary tumors at *B* and *C* and carcinoma in the pectoral muscle at *A*. (Reprinted from Wainwright [23]. By permission of Surgery, Gynecology & Obstetrics.)

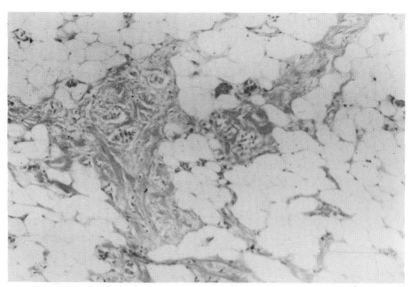

FIG. 9. Cancer removed by simple mastectomy; note involvement of deep fascia.

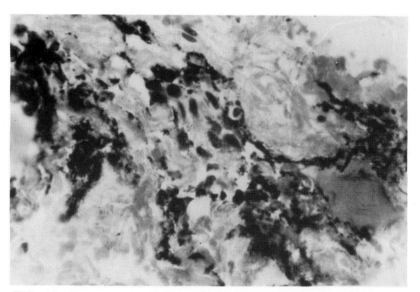

FIG. 10. Cancer removed by radical mastectomy. India ink staining delineates the levels of muscle and pectoralis fasica; note tumor below these levels.

In the same vein, Figure 11 presents the decreasing incidence of radical procedures at our institution, a trend that has occurred throughout the country. In this graph, one can see that the incidence of radical mastectomy, as indicated by the hatched lines, has been decreasing steadily. In the five-year period of 1974 through 1978, the number of patients undergoing radical mastectomy is practically halved. On the other hand, modified radical mastectomies have steadily increased. Of interest also is the fact that the incidence of invasive duct carcinoma is fairly constant, between 70% and 80%. These figures are similar to the figures in most large institutions and represent the preponderance of malignancies that we are seeing. It is apparent that, without even going into the specifics of extension of these lesions, whether they are early or late, there must be a disproportionate number of lesser procedures being done for invasive cancer. This is a trend that I fear, because if it is occurring in our institution, it must also be occurring in other institutions and even more so in community hospitals. It is obvious that surgeons are doing simple procedures across the

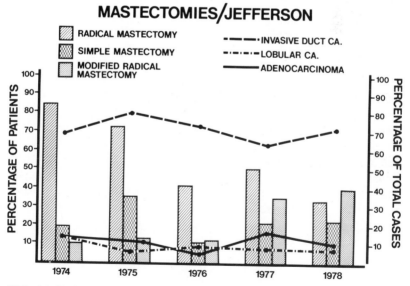

FIG. 11. Incidence of various types of mastectomies performed at Thomas Jefferson University Hospital from 1974 to 1978.

board without sufficient selectivity and knowledge of the histology or the extent of the lesion.

It is very difficult to accept a deviation from the standard surgical method of treatment of breast carcinoma for invasive carcinoma, which would be en bloc dissection of the primary tumor and the lymphatics. I know of no area except cancer surgery in which this concept is violated. What responsible surgeon would resect a carcinoma of the colon, trying explicitly to remove all of the aortic nodes while leaving the mesentery? This to me is very similar to the procedure advocated in modified radical mastectomy.

In summary, I have presented one surgeon's opinion about a complex situation that we face in the treatment of breast carcinoma. I have specifically avoided entering into a statistical analysis of various studies related to lesser procedures vs. radical mastectomy, because I feel they prove nothing. I have tried to point out the specific areas of contention that exist between the two schools of thought for breast carcinoma. There is no optimum treatment yet. We do not use the word "cure" in discussing breast carcinoma; rather, we use the word "survival." Until we obtain methods of determining the presence of systemic disease — and so far this is not distinguishable by routine ancillary testing — or we are provided with a method of treating systemic disease with the hope of cure, it is my belief that patients with invasive breast carcinoma who fall within the realm of operability should be subjected to adequate and thorough radical mastectomy. If regional nodal involvement is demonstrated or medial quadrant lesions are present, postoperative radiation therapy should be administered. It is possible that we also will be treating individuals who *probably* could be cured by lesser procedures. Unfortunately, at present we cannot determine who these individuals are. Therefore, in trying to serve all of our patients to the best of our ability and offering them the best possible chance for longer survival, radical mastectomy and radiation therapy, when indicated, are my personal choices for treatment.

References

1. Moore, C.H.: On the influence of inadequate operations on the theory of cancer. Roy. Med. Chir. Soc. (Lond.) 1:245, 1867.

2. Banks, W.M.: Some Results of the Operative Treatment of Cancer of the Breast. Edinburgh:Niell & Co., 1882, p. 16.
3. Gross, S.W.: Tumors of the Mammary Gland. New York:D. Appleton & Co., 1880.
4. Qualhein, R.E. and Gall, E.A.: Breast carcinoma with multiple sites of origin. Cancer 10:460-468, 1957.
5. Stewart, H.J., cited by Forrest, A.P.M.: Management of early carcinoma of the breast. Proc. Roy. Soc. Med. 63:107-110, 1970.
6. Morganstern, L., Kaufman, P.A. and Friedman, N.B.: The case against tylectomy for carcinoma of the breast: The factor of multicentricity. Am. J. Surg. 130:251-258, 1975.
7. Gallagher, H.S. and Martin, J.C.: The study of mammary carcinoma and whole organ sectioning. Cancer 23:855-873, 1969.
8. Berger, S.M., Gershon-Cohen, J. and Beherend, A.: The earlier diagnosis of breast carcinoma. Arch. Surg. 86:150-154, 1963.
9. Millis, R.R. and Thynne, S.J.: In-situ intraductal carcinoma of the breast: A long term follow-up study. Br. J. Surg. 62:957-962, 1975.
10. Moskowitz, M., Sheshagiriroo, P., Fidlen, J.A. et al: The diagnosis of minimal breast cancer in a screened population. Cancer 37:2543-2552, 1976.
11. Westbrook, K.C. and Gallagher, H.S.: Intraductal carcinoma of the breast. Am. J. Surg. 130:667-670, 1975.
12. Barker, W.F., Sperling, L., Dowdy, A.H. et al: Management of nonpalpable breast carcinoma discovered by mammography. Ann. Surg. 50:385-394, 1969.
13. Frankl, G. and Rosenfeld, D.D.: Xeroradiographic detection of occult breast cancer. Cancer 35:542-548, 1975.
14. Malone, L.J., Frankl, G., Dorazio, R. and Winkly, J.H.: Occult breast cancer detected by xeroradiography: Clinical consideration. Ann. Surg. 181:133-136, 1975.
15. Strax, P.: Results in mass screening for breast cancer in young women. Am. J. Surg. 129:289-291, 1975.
16. Dowdy, A.H., Barker, W.F., Lagosse, L.D. et al: Mammography as a screening method for the examination of large populations. Cancer 28:1558-1562, 1971.
17. Shapiro, S., Strax, P. and Venet, L.: Periodic breast cancer screening in reducing mortality from breast cancer. JAMA 215:1777-1785, 1971.
18. Byrd, B.F.: Breast cancer: Has the tide turned? Breast 2:23-25, 1976.
19. Pickren, J.W.: Significance of occult metastasis. Cancer 14:1266, 1961.
20. Saphir, O. and Amromin, G.D.: Obscure lymph node metastasis in carcinoma of the breast. Cancer 1:238, 1948.
21. Hultborn, A., Hulten, I., Roos, B. et al: Evaluation of regional lymph drainage from mammary gland and hand to the axillary nodes. Acta Radiol. Ther. Phys. Biol. 9:489, 1970.
22. Caceres, E., Lingan, M. and Gelgado, P.: Evaluation of dissection of the axilla in modified radical mastectomy. Surg. Gynecol. Obstet. 143:395, 1976.

23. Wainwright, J.M.: Muscle involvement in breast cancer. Surg. Gynecol. Obstet. 52:549, 1931.

Self-Evaluation Quiz

1. Modified radical mastectomy is the operation of choice in most cancers of the breast because lymphatics do not pass through the pectoralis muscles.
   a) True
   b) False
2. There is no difference in the ten-year survival figures in most large series in compared modified mastectomies and radical mastectomies.
   a) True
   b) False
3. All lymph nodes anatomically present in patients with breast carcinoma can be readily removed with the modified radical procedure.
   a) True
   b) False
4. The "minimal carcinoma" is a lesion which lends itself more readily to the modified surgical procedures because there is practically never lymph node involvement.
   a) True
   b) False
5. Despite the fact that the incidence of invasive ductal carcinoma has remained constant over the last five years, the number of radical surgical procedures for carcinoma of the breast has decreased markedly.
   a) True
   b) False

Answers on page 335.

Lumpectomy and Irradiation as an Alternative to Mastectomy in Early Carcinoma of the Breast

Peggie Ann Findlay, M.D. and Robert L. Goodman, M.D.

Objectives

The optimal treatment for early breast cancer remains controversial. The history of our understanding of the biology of breast carcinoma and evolution of treatment philosophy are reviewed. The emergence of limited surgery and radical irradiation as an alternative to radical surgery is examined. Current recommendations for treatment are discussed.

The changing concept of tumor biology and the development of new treatment modalities necessitate reappraisal of current standard therapy of early breast carcinoma. Growth of sophistication in all oncologic specialties now offers some patients equivalent probability of cure with avoidance of physical deformity and its concomitant psychological trauma.

Ionizing radiation has been used with increasing effectiveness as an anticancer agent since the year following Roentgen's discovery of x-rays. There are abundant data for a variety of tumor sites and types to indicate that doses of 4400 to 5000 rads in 4½ to 5 weeks have an excellent probability of achieving sterilization of microscopic disease, and that doses of 6600 to 7000 rads in 6½ to 7 weeks are effective in sterilizing small volumes of gross disease [1]. These observations, coupled with good preservation of normal functional anatomy, make primary

Peggie Ann Findlay, M.D., Resident; and Robert L. Goodman, M.D., Professor and Chairman, Departments of Radiation Therapy at the University of Pennsylvania School of Medicine and the Fox Chase Cancer Center, Philadelphia.

radiation therapy the treatment of choice in many carcinomas of the head, neck, prostate and uterine cervix. It is hardly surprising that comparable doses have been found to be equally effective in the treatment of breast cancer [2-4].

During the last 15 years, the concept of the natural history of breast cancer has changed dramatically. The idea that the tumor grew locally, then spread in a predictable fashion to regional lymph nodes and later metastasized hematogenously to distant sites underlay the Halstedian principles of large en bloc resection. Throughout the first half of the century, a variety of local procedures was proposed in order to sterilize local disease and thereby improve cure; but in trial after trial, even with such procedures as the extended radical mastectomy, survival stage for stage was depressingly consistent and highly correlated with axillary node status. Among patients with apparently localized disease at initial therapy, 25% of node-negative and more than 75% of node-positive patients were dead of breast cancer in ten years [5-10] (Table 1). In addition, those patients who did not receive en bloc resections seemed to fare no worse [11]. Fisher was one of the first to recognize and stress that breast cancer at the time of clinical presentation is a systemic disease; others later came to recognize that nodal metastases are an indicator of the host-tumor relationship and imply disseminated disease in a high proportion of patients [12]. The development of effective adjuvant chemotherapy directed against micrometastasis is likely to impact favorably on ultimate survival [13]. In accordance with this new philosophy, a less radical procedure that offers a high

Table 1. Breast Cancer Survival: Radical Surgery

Author	Treatment*	Neg. Axilla, % Survival	No. Patients Evaluable	Pos. Axilla, % Survival	No. Patients Evaluable	Years of Follow-up
Easson [6]	RM ± XRT	70	(526)	35	(931)	10
Valagussa [7]	RM ± ERM	72	(335)	24	(381)	10
NSABP [5]	RM ± XRT	77	(159)	48	(269)	5
Urban [8]	ERM	72	(144)	37	(171)	10
Donegan [9]	RM	74	(332)	30	(456)	10
Haagensen [10]	RM	75	(484)	42	(398)	10

*RM = radical mastectomy; ERM = extended radical mastectomy; XRT = radiation therapy.

probability of local control is feasible, with the addition of adjuvant chemotherapy in node-positive patients. This technique has the potential to become a standard treatment in early breast cancer, at least in those centers with sufficient technical capabilities.

Traditionally, radiation therapy has played an adjuvant role in the management of breast cancer. Over the years it has been delivered pre- or post-operatively in combination with a variety of surgical procedures. The heated controversy which raged for so long over the best surgical procedure, with or without the addition of radiation therapy, is finally being laid to rest by the emergence of effective chemotherapy. In principle, however, the addition of radiation to surgery has not been advocated as superior in terms of survival by most radiotherapists. The National Surgical Adjuvant Breast Project in 1970 published the results of a prospective randomized trial of women with operable breast cancer [5]. Patients were randomized after conventional radical mastectomy to receive postoperative radiotherapy, consisting of 3500 rads in three weeks to 4500 rads in five weeks to the internal mammary nodes, axillary apex and supraclavicular region only (470 patients); three days of thiotepa (316 patients); or placebo (317 patients). Analysis at 1½, 3 and 5 years showed no significant differences in survival. However, regional failure, defined as reappearance of disease within the radiated volume, at 5 years was 0.6% in the radiotherapy group vs. 8.5% of placebo and 3.8% of thiotepa patients. Easson published ten-year results of the Manchester trials [6]. Following radical mastectomy, 752 patients were randomized to receive no further therapy until recurrence ("watched" group), while 961 patients received postoperative x-ray therapy by one of two techniques. Again there was no difference in ultimate survival, although overall incidence of local failure at ten years was reduced from 32% in the watched to 19% in the treated patients. Ultimate control of local disease, however, was equivalent with overall incidence of local disease persisting at death, i.e. 14% in the treated group vs. 16% in the watched patients. Numerous other studies have confirmed these observations [14]. It would appear that the development of adjuvant chemotherapy has made most of the traditional considerations for postoperative radiation therapy obsolete, at least in clinical stages I and II [13]. Our current recommendations for postoperative radiotherapy in this group are limited and individualized to those patients at an extremely high risk of local failure, e.g. positive margins of resection and extension of tumor into axillary fat.

An issue may emerge in the future concerning a very select group of patients and the role of postoperative irradiation. There is a suggestion in several studies [7, 8, 15] that the small group of patients with medial or central lesions and positive axillary nodes may be benefited, in terms of survival, by treatment of the internal mammary node chain by irradiation or surgical removal. After adjuvant chemotherapy has been more thoroughly evaluated, this question may deserve further study.

Radiation therapy as a primary modality in breast cancer has a surprisingly long history. Geoffry Keynes reported in 1929 [16] and 1937 [17] his results with interstitial radium. He achieved five-year survival of 71% in 75 patients with disease confined to the breast, and 29% in 66 patients with apparent axillary involvement. Recognizing the difficulty in controlling large tumors, he later modified his regimen to include excisional biopsy of bulky masses. Baclesse [18] from the Foundation Curie published a remarkable article in 1949 reviewing his results of primary radiation, using what we would now consider to be primitive external beam equipment (180 KV, 1-mm Cu filter). All of the 130 treated patients would today be considered to have advanced local disease. Not only did he achieve a 31.5% three-year disease-free overall survival, but he also documented control as a function of dose and greater degree of tissue tolerance with prolonged fractionation.

Over the last quarter-century, increasing numbers of institutions have reported their experiences with radical radiotherapy [19-25]. Initial interest was centered in Europe but more recently several American groups have become active. Specific techniques of radiotherapy have differed, as has the preceding surgical procedure. This has ranged from incisional biopsy (Paris) to wedge mastectomy (Toronto). Some patients in the last few years have also received adjuvant chemotherapy. The studies are generally single-institution and nonrandomized, and, in addition, these series are small. The NSABP, Milan group and the NIH have all instituted prospective randomized trials which are currently in progress [26, 27]. However, a review of the collection of representative data (Table 2) is quite instructive.

A new form of therapy must meet two criteria. First, local control and ultimate survival must be at least equivalent to results of the standard treatment. In addition, the cosmetic result must be significantly superior.

It seems clear from evaluation of available data that minimal surgery followed by irradiation can meet the first criterion mentioned above. It appears that the technique from the Joint Center of Radiation Therapy [22] of lumpectomy, external irradiation and boost iridium implant can result in a local-regional failure of less than 7% in clinical stage I and II disease. The higher rate of local failure reported in the two French series [24, 25], in which incisional biopsy only was performed for tumor masses greater than 3 cm, can almost certainly be attributed to the presence of bulky disease at the initiation of radiation therapy. It is important to note, however, that ultimate survival at ten years may not be significantly worsened in these instances. Apparently the French school bases its practice on the belief that good cosmesis cannot be achieved after removal of a large lump. It must be pointed out, though, that the deformed fibrotic breast seen after the high dose necessary to eradicate such disease, or the defect left by subsequent surgery, cannot be considered cosmetically ideal. In fact, excellent cosmesis can readily be achieved after excision of T2 and even selected T3 tumors.

Complications of technically meticulous radiation therapy have been minimal. They consist of occasional lymphedema of the arm and/or breast (occurring almost exclusively in conjunction with extensive axillary node dissection), radiation pneumonitis and rib fractures.

As this technique becomes more widely used, several issues are likely to emerge. The question of the necessity of a boost dose to the tumor bed or the type of boost will need to be answered. Several methods are currently available for delivering such a boost. These consist of small fields delivered with external or electron beam, or interstitial implantation. All three can be delivered with negligible morbidity. An interstitial implant can be performed under local anesthesia but requires

Table 2. Breast Cancer Survival and Local Recurrence: Limited Surgery with Radical Irradiation

Author	No. Patients	Treatment	AJC Stage	No. of Patients Surviving/No. at Risk	% Survival	% Local Recurrence
Proznitz [19]	150	L + XRT	I	46/49	91*	6.6 overall
			II	75/101	60	
Alpert [20]	49	XRT ± L	T1	16/18	††	8 overall
			T2	22/26		
			T3	4/5		
Peters [21]	184	WR + XRT		20-Year survival – 50% in both groups		
	552	RM + XRT		Local recurrence – 7.8% (WR + XRT)		
Hellman [22]	176	L + XRT	I	62	96*	5
			II	122	68	7
RTOG [23]	234	XRT ± L/WR	I	112	83*	1.7
			II	112	68	9.7 with excision
						29.2 no excision
Calle [24]	514	L + XRT if <3 cm	T <3 cm	102/120	85‡	13
		XRT alone if ≥3 cm	T >3 cm	268/394	68	59
Pierquin [25]	177	L + XRT if <3 cm	T1	36/43	84‡	4.5
		XRT alone if ≥3 cm	T2	72/91	79	7.5
			T3	24/43	56	23

L = lumpectomy; WR = wedge resection; RM = radical mastectomy; XRT = radiation therapy.
*Five-year actuarial NED.
†Minimum two-year, average four-year follow-up survival NED.
‡Five-year absolute survival.

hospitalization. The availability of particular equipment and the cosmetic results achieved by different techniques will probably be important considerations in the final treatment recommendations.

Perhaps more important will be the impact of systemic chemotherapy on local control. In Bonadonna's initial report of CMF chemotherapy as adjuvant treatment following radical mastectomy in patients with primary breast cancer and positive axillary nodes [13], the incidence of local-regional failure was 9.4% in 179 control patients as compared to 1.9% of 207 CMF patients. If these results are confirmed with further follow-up and in other institutions, it may be possible to reduce the treatment volume in node-positive patients treated with both radical radiation and adjuvant chemotherapy.

At the University of Pennsylvania, we have adopted a fairly comprehensive treatment policy in identifying and treating patients who may be candidates for radical radiotherapy. The most important consideration is the patient's own preference. While most patients would much prefer to retain their breasts, there are some who would suffer continuing anxiety should the cancerous breast not be removed. A few would rather undergo a less time-consuming and inconvenient procedure.

If the patient desires an alternative to mastectomy, an initial evaluation consisting of complete history and physical examination, with detailed description of both breasts, breast mass, and axillary and supraclavicular contents, is mandatory. It is preferable to have the radiotherapist examine the patient before excision. IUCC/AJC stage T1, T2, N0, N1 disease [28] (Table 3) is acceptable unless the breast is so small in relation to tumor size that lumpectomy itself would leave a cosmetically deformed breast. Metastatic work-up, including CBC, liver function tests, chest x-ray and bone scan, must be negative. Preoperative bilateral mammograms are obtained. Patients are rejected if mammograms show excessively large, diffuse or multifocal disease as evidenced by diffuse microcalcifications. In our institution, such criteria have excluded approximately 10% of evaluated clinical stage I and II patients.

Surgery is then performed, consisting of excision of gross disease. It is not necessary to obtain a wide margin of resection. On the contrary, the smallest possible amount of tissue that

Table 3. Staging of Breast Cancer

Primary Tumor
- T1 — Tumor 2 cm or less in greatest dimension
- T2 — Tumor greater than 2 cm but no more than 5 cm in greatest dimension
- T3 — Tumor more than 5 cm in greatest dimension
- T4 — Tumor of any size with direct extension to chest wall or skin

Nodal Involvement
- N0 — No palpable homolateral axillary nodes
- N1 — Movable homolateral axillary nodes
  - N1a — Nodes not considered to contain growth
  - N1b — Nodes considered to contain growth
- N2 — Homolateral axillary nodes containing growth and fixed to one another or to other structures
- N3 — Homolateral supraclavicular or infraclavicular nodes containing growth, or edema of the arm

Distant Metastases
- M0 — No known distant metastasis
- M1 — Distant metastasis present

Stage Grouping
Stage I
    T1, N0 or N1a, M0

Stage II
    T1, N1b, M0
    T2, N0 or N1a or N1b, M0

Stage III
    Any T3, N1 or N2, M0

Stage IV
    T4, Any N, Any M
    Any T, N3, Any M
    Any T, Any N, M1

includes the mass is taken in order to achieve the best cosmetic results. At the same time, sampling of level I axillary nodes is obtained. Results of the examination of these nodes are considered in radiation therapy treatment planning, as determinants in treating the patient with adjuvant chemotherapy and as an indicator of ultimate prognosis. If the patient is of an age and medical condition where adjuvant chemotherapy cannot be administered, axillary sampling is omitted in clinical N0 patients. Estrogen receptors are obtained on the pathologic specimen. Ten days to two weeks is then allotted for healing.

Axillary sampling rather than full axillary dissection is being evaluated at the University of Pennsylvania in order to reduce the incidence of posttherapy lymphedema of the breast and arm [29]. The median number of nodes removed is 8 (range 2 to 23). Of 66 T1, T2, N0, N1, M0 patients, 20 (30%) were found to have nodal involvement. This percentage compares well with expected results in axillary dissection. Despite suggestive reports from other institutions [30, 31], it is too early to make definite conclusions regarding the role of sampling vs. formal dissection.

Radiation treatment planning is then begun. Areas irradiated depend on the position of the tumor in the breast and on the results of the axillary sampling. If the disease is in the outer quadrant of the breast and the axillary sampling is negative, we do not irradiate either the internal mammary, axillary or supraclavicular regions. If the axillary sampling is negative, but the disease is in the inner or central quadrants, we again do not radiate the axilla or supraclavicular areas; however, we do attempt to treat the internal mammary nodes. If the axillary sampling produces positive results, we radiate all the nodal draining areas (Table 4). The only deviation in this policy is in those patients with outer quadrant disease and positive axillae who have large, pendulous breasts or a thoracic cavity contour that prohibits adequate treatment. In these we elect not to treat the internal mammary nodes in order to reduce the amount of lung in the irradiated field. The use of an en face internal mammary field is possible, but it causes potential problems of over- or under-dosage in the inner quadrant of the treated breast and may produce inferior cosmesis.

The patient receives 4400 to 5000 rads to the entire breast and internal mammary nodes (if included in the treatment

Table 4. Treatment Areas in Addition to Breast
by Quadrant and Axillary Node Status

	Axilla −	*Axilla* +
Outer quadrant	None	All nodal draining areas
Inner or central quadrant	Internal mammary nodes	All nodal draining areas

volume) by opposing wedged tangential fields. This technique assures a homogenous dose distribution throughout the treatment volume. As the skin of the breast is not felt to be at risk, and cosmesis would be compromised, the use of bolus is avoided. The axilla and supraclavicular area is treated by an anterior field, angled off the spinal cord, at 200 rads a day to a dose of 4400 to 4600 rads to a depth of 5 cm. This dose is occasionally supplemented by a posterior axillary boost field. Ten days to two weeks after the external irradiation is completed, the patient undergoes implantation, usually under local anesthesia. The implant is individualized with regard to breast size and initial tumor size. A dose of 1500 to 2000 rads is delivered to the implanted volume over 45 to 55 hours. The isotope used in iridium 192. The patient is seen in routine follow-up, with mammograms obtained yearly and blood counts and chest x-rays as indicated.

Depending on the axillary nodal status, adjuvant chemotherapy is administered. The regimen used presently is CMFP (cyclophosphamide, methotrexate, 5-fluorouracil, prednisone). Because of recent data indicating that postmenopausal patients who receive full doses of drug show the same response to adjuvant chemotherapy as premenopausal patients, drugs are prescribed without regard to menopausal status [32]. It is also felt that early exposure to the drug is important [33]. Full-dose Cytoxan and 5-FU are started at the initiation of x-ray therapy, and methotrexate and prednisone are added after completion. Twelve cycles of full CMFP are delivered.

Certainly, a number of issues remain concerning radical irradiation as an alternative to mastectomy in early breast cancer. In particular, the amount of breast tissue removed, the necessity for and type of boost dose, the extent of axillary surgery and the influence of chemotherapy on local control are presently undergoing evaluation. However, it is our feeling that the local control following lumpectomy, axillary sampling and radical irradiation is so high that in selected centers this procedure is a viable alternative to radical surgery.

References

1. Fletcher, G.H.: Clinical dose response curves of human malignant epithelial tumors. Br. J. Radiol. 46:1-12, 1973.

2. Fletcher, G.H.: Local results of irradiation in the primary management of localized breast cancer. Cancer 29:545-551, 1972.
3. Ghossein, N.A., Stacey, P., Alpert, S. et al: Local control of breast cancer with tumorectomy plus radiotherapy or radiotherapy alone. Radiology 121:455-459, 1976.
4. Montague, E.D., Gutierrez, A.E., Barker, J.L. et al: Conservation surgery and irradiation for the treatment of favorable breast cancer. Cancer 43:1058-1061, 1979.
5. Fisher, B., Slack, N.H., Cavanaugh, P.J. et al: Postoperative radiotherapy in the treatment of breast cancer: Results of the NSABP clinical trial. Ann. Surg. 172:711-732, 1978.
6. Easson, E.C.: Post-operative radiotherapy and breast cancer. In Prognostic Factors in Breast Cancer. Edinburgh:J. & S. Livingstone, 1968, pp. 118-127.
7. Valagussa, P., Bonadonna, G. and Veronesi, U.: Patterns of relapse and survival following radical mastectomy. Cancer 41:1170-1178, 1978.
8. Urban, J. and Castro, E.B.: Selecting variations in extent of surgical procedure for breast cancer. Cancer 28:1615-1623, 1971.
9. Donegan, W.L.: The influence of untreated internal mammary metastasis upon the course of mammary cancer. Cancer 39:533-538, 1977.
10. Haagensen, C.D.: In Diseases of the Breast. Philadelphia:W. B. Saunders Co., 1971, pp. 704-734.
11. Fisher, B., Montague, E., Redmond, C. et al: Comparison of radical mastectomy with alternative treatments for primary breast cancer: A first report of results from a prospective randomized clinical trial. Cancer 39:2827-2839, 1977.
12. Fisher, B.: Breast cancer management: Alternatives to radical mastectomy, editorial. N. Eng. J. Med. 301:326-328, 1979.
13. Bonadonna, G., Brusamolino, E., Valagussa, P. et al: Combination chemotherapy as an adjuvant treatment in operable breast cancer. N. Engl. J. Med. 294:405-410, 1976.
14. Stewart, H.J.: Controlled trials in the treatment of "early" breast cancer: A review of published results. World J. Surg. 1:309-313, 1977.
15. Høst, H. and Brennhovd, I.: The effect of post-operative radiotherapy in breast cancer. Int. J. Rad. Oncol. Biol. Phys. 2:1061-1067, 1977.
16. Keynes, G.: The treatment of primary carcinoma of the breast with radium. Acta Radiol. 10:393-402, 1929.
17. Keynes, G.: Conservative treatment of cancer of the breast. Br. Med. J. 2:643-647, 1937.
18. Baclesse, S.: Roentgen therapy as the sole method of treatment of cancer of the breast. Am. J. Roent. 62:311-319, 1949.
19. Proznitz, L.R., Goldenberg, I.S., Packard, R.A. et al: Radiation therapy as initial treatment for early stage cancer of the breast without mastectomy. Cancer 39:917-923, 1977.
20. Alpert, S., Ghossein, N.A., Stacey, P. et al: Primary management of operable breast cancer by minimal surgery and radiotherapy. Cancer 42:2054-2058, 1978.

21. Peters, M.V.: Cutting the Gordian Knot in early breast cancer. Ann. R. Coll. Phys. Surg. Can. 8:186-192, 1975.

22. Harris, J., Levene, M. and Hellman, S.: The role of radiation therapy in the primary treatment of carcinoma of the breast. Semin. Oncol. 5:403-416, 1978.

23. Bedwinek, J.M., Perez, C.A., Kramer, S. et al: Irradiation as the primary management of stage I and II adenocarcinoma of the breast: Analysis of the RTOG breast registry. Cancer Clin. Trials 3:11-18, 1980.

24. Calle, R., Pilleron, J.P., Schlienger, P. and Vileoq, J.R.: Conservative management of operable breast cancer: 10 Years experience of the Foundation Curie. Cancer 42:2045-2053, 1978.

25. Pierquin, B., Owen, R., Maylin, C. et al: Radical radiation therapy of breast cancer. Int. J. Radiat. Oncol. Biol. Phys. 6:17-24, 1980.

26. Veronesi, V.: Conservation treatment of breast cancer: A trial in progress at the Cancer Institute of Milan. World J. Surg. 1:324-236, 1977.

27. Fisher, B.: United States trials of conservative surgery. World J. Surg. 1:327-335, 1977.

28. Manual for Staging of Cancer. American Joint Committee for Cancer Staging and End Results Reporting, 1977.

29. Richter, M.P., Carabell, S.C., Bryan, J.H. et al: The role of axillary sampling in the primary radiation therapy of primary breast cancer. Proc. Am. Soc. Clin. Oncol. 21:414, 1980.

30. Forrest, A.P.M., Roberts, M.M., Cant, E.L.M. et al: Simple mastectomy and pectoral node biopsy: The Cardiff-St. Mary's trial. World J. Surg. 1:320-323, 1977.

31. Bluming, A.Z., Ozohan, M.L., Marks, R. et al: Lumpectomy, radical axillary node dissection, external beam radiotherapy and iridium implant as treatment of primary breast cancer — A community based study. Proc. Am. Soc. Clin. Oncol. 21:405, 1980.

32. Bonadonna, G. and Valagussa, P.: Dose response effect of CMF in breast cancer. Proc. Am. Soc. Clin. Oncol. 21:413, 1980.

33. Nissen-Meyer, R.: One short chemotherapy course in primary breast cancer: 12 Year follow-up in series 1 of the Scandinavian Adjuvant Chemotherapy Study Group. In Jones, S.E. and Salmon, S.E. (eds.): Adjuvant Therapy of Cancer II. New York:Grune & Stratton, 1979, pp. 297-213.

Self-Evaluation Quiz

1. Breast cancer:
   a) Grows locally, then spreads predictably to regional lymph nodes and later metastasizes hematogenously to distant sites
   b) Is often a systemic disease at clinical presentation
2. In most patients treated with radical surgery, the addition

of postoperative radiotherapy:
a) Increases ultimate survival
b) Decreases ultimate survival
c) Decreases local recurrence

3. Metastases to axillary lymph nodes are only an indication of advanced local disease in most patients.
a) True
b) False

4. Radiation therapy as a primary treatment modality in early breast cancer is a recent development.
a) True
b) False

5. Local control of the primary tumor by radiotherapy is probably influenced by:
a) The presence of bulky disease at initiation of therapy
b) The total dose delivered
c) Technique of therapy
d) All of the above

6. The advantage of lumpectomy and radical irradiation over radical surgery in the treatment of early breast cancer is:
a) Improved survival
b) Improved cosmesis
c) Both a and b

7. All patients with T1 and T2 breast lesions are candidates for lumpectomy and radical radiotherapy.
a) True
b) False

8. Information obtained from pathologic examination of axillary lymph nodes is used:
a) In radiation treatment planning
b) To determine candidates for adjuvant chemotherapy
c) As a prognostic indicator
d) All of the above

9. When performing lumpectomy prior to radical irradiation, it is important to obtain a wide margin of normal tissue around the mass.
a) True
b) False

10. Because of the toxicity of some chemotherapeutic agents when combined with radiation, chemotherapy in node-

positive patients is delayed until radiotherapy is completed.
a) True
b) False

Answers on page 335.

Physician-Patient Responsibility in Breast Cancer Management: The Value of Patient Participation

Wendy S. Schain, Ed.D.

Objectives

The intent of this paper is to promote a more egalitarian relationship in health care and to suggest reasons why patient participation should be encouraged. Several general guidelines are presented and a basic theoretical model to anchor these perceptions is described. In addition, specific recommendations about what not to say are recorded, along with clear suggestions about verbal prescriptions which are inherent in a high-quality interaction between doctor and patient.

Introduction: Medicine Is a Consumer Item

The lay person's naivete and lack of responsible behavior exhibited in health care is not so evident in any other consumer purchase. Women who want to buy a major household item such as a refrigerator, washing machine or microwave oven often research the product thoroughly and "shop" around to find the best buy and the most reliable service for the investment they are about to make. A skillful sales person may motivate the purchaser to select a more expensive model or in some way upgrade her choice, but in general, the ultimate decision rests with the purchaser. This careful investigative process and guided search for the right buy is glaringly absent in

---

Wendy S. Schain, Ed.D., Medical Care Consultant, National Institutes of Health, Clinical Center, Bethesda, Md.

the selection of medical service. Often when a woman is faced with the need for a doctor, or specifically with the need for a specialist (e.g. surgical oncologist), she lets another person or physician make that decision. Many times the ultimate choices about what doctor to consult, what hospital to go to and what treatment really is best for her particular condition are decided without her engaging in serious dialogue or research about existing alternatives. In general, women lack clear-cut guidelines and knowledge about what to ask for regarding the competence and experience of the involved physician and/or the benefits vs. risks of the treatment recommended. Too often women are more critical and demanding about the qualifications of their hairdressers and household help than they are of the persons to whom they go for the healing of their bodies or their psyches.

Many women choose their physicians in a kind of random fashion, because he/she practices in a convenient location, is married to a friend, was recommended by a clergyman or was a classmate in school. Lay people are not taught how to systematically choose and evaluate medical services, so the events which transpire often are left, in part, up to fate. In addition, some of the seductions of the Madison Avenue world of advertising also enter into the decisions and purchase incentives which influence medical care options. Reports of good outcome in popular magazines, stories about successful healing from nontraditional therapies, community publicity about Dr. X's reputation all combine to stimulate choice. These motivational factors, however, originate from outside the person, and the individual patient is still left without a clear set of internalized criteria to make important decisions. What seems essential from this set of circumstances is to recognize that society has an obligation to educate the public about factors crucial to the purchase of medical services. Patients need to learn to enter the marketplace of medical care with a standard set of intelligent questions and the feeling that they have the right to ask for information about a physician's qualifications, experience with certain procedures (e.g. modified radical mastectomy) and the effects of accepting or refusing certain treatments. This paper, therefore, will attempt to describe contemporary causes of this inequitable condition in medical care, as well as the motivating forces currently operating to bring about more patient participation with a higher level of informed consumerism.

The Notion of Aesculapian Authority

Until recently, decisions about patient care belonged solely to the realm of the physician with very little weight or credence being given to the opinions of the patient. Advances in legal, ethical and moral attitudes in health care over the last two decades, however, have skyrocketed a major interest in self-determination and patient rights. Therefore, it has become essential to examine the physician-patient interaction and to uncover the dynamics by which this relationship influences the individual patient and impacts the decisions she makes about her treatments and the quality of her life. Today's lay person is beginning to recognize that the purchase of medical services is a major consumer activity — one that requires new awareness of substantive information as well as the acquisition of certain assertive behaviors. Patients are actively becoming more involved in their own health care and are developing skills to assist them in making correct decisions about what type of doctor should treat them, how to evaluate the risks-benefits of certain therapies and, most important, how to communicate to their physicians about certain needs and anxieties they may harbor.

The obvious lack of parity between a physician and his/her patient is part of a cultural trend which was conceived and perpetrated by the concept of "aesculapian authority." This notion implies that the physician has the ultimate power and should be regarded as the unchallenged decision maker in health planning. Such a view of unilateral authority residing with the doctor puts the patient in a very dependent position and fosters the belief that only the physician has the power to heal. In addition, such prevailing attitudes have stimulated the feeling that doctors are mystical, and regard for them sometimes crosses over into idolatry. Some patients believe that their doctor's title, "M.D.," stands for "Minor Deity," wherein the physician has a magic connection to the spiritual forces that affect life and death. In addition, the laity imagines that the physician's acceptance of the Hippocratic Oath establishes him/her as a great humanitarian whose major commitment is to serve the best interests of his/her patient population. Because the aesculapian concept "... does not dispose (one) toward sharing information about diagnostic studies, treatment approaches, prognoses and other data with the patient" [1], it is no wonder that most of the communication in health care has been a one-way dialogue. Patients in general, and women in particular, have been quite reluctant to contest statements made by their doctor, voice their own opinions or request information that would require the attending physician to give supporting evidence for his recommendation. The balance of power in medical practice is shifting now, and patients are becoming more involved and vocal about their own self-interest and the role they wish to play in the decisions regarding their health care.

A New Emphasis in Medicine: The Doctor-Patient Relationship

Behavioral science has helped to shift our focus away from just examining the outcome of treatment to exploring the dynamics of the physician-patient interaction and the significant influence this interaction has on the patient's decision making, reports of satisfaction with care and perhaps even adherence to medical regimens. The expanded awareness of the impact of the personal ingredient on health care demands a reappraisal of models of patient-physician interreaction in an effort to understand the costs-benefits associated with different levels of patient participation. Women in general, and breast cancer patients in particular, are demonstrating their increased interest in assuming responsibility for their health care, the treatments recommended to them, their quality of life and even the quality of their dying [2]. This change in standard procedures makes it necessary to suggest some alterations in shaping contemporary attitudes of practitioners as well as in defining goals of medical school education. It has become essential to teach patients to acquire appropriate consumer behaviors to secure qualified medical care, and at the same time to encourage physicians to recognize the therapeutic value that this patient activism will provide.

Until recently, most physician-patient transactions did not

contain a large dose of serious dialogue or exchange of feelings as part of the delivery of services. The right to voice opinions, make recommendations and express value judgments had been the primary responsibility of the physician, with only minimal regard given to the requests of the patient. This paternalistic model of health care, which carried with it the image of patients as unquestioning, malleable, child-like figures, is being replaced by a more humanitarian and egalitarian paradigm that values reciprocity of communication. The formerly held aesculapian authority model expected a patient to comply without inquiry and to be happy with whatever participation was permitted. It did not, however, take into account the important influences of psychological and transactional factors in reports of satisfaction with medical care and the patient's actual compliance with treatment regimens. Interestingly, patient compliance has been positively correlated with the expression of warmth and concern on the part of the physician and an impression of free exchange of information between the two parties [3]. Acknowledging that these conditions exert such strong influences on patient response, academicians will undoubtedly mold plans for revised educational programming for physicians which will include critical factors that have been overlooked for too long. Two of the most pressing considerations will be to give attention to (1) the seriousness of the patient's need to be involved in what is going to happen to him/her, and (2) the value that patient participation has on the individual's overall satisfaction with care and response to treatment. The key element seems to be involvement on the part of the patient and support (not coercion) as the response from the physician.

Unfortunately, this type of equitable alliance between doctor and patient has not been fashionable or publicly supported. In fact, such an interchange would have been viewed as highly suspect by the medical profession. A lucid illustration of how new and unfamiliar is this notion of reciprocal alliance or *shared responsibility* in medicine is reflected in the following discourse between two practicing physicians regarding the issue of future medical school education [4]:

> Of all the things this panel can do to help Dr. Everyman, the most important, I believe, is to convince him of the value of concerted effort to give patients what they want. I

think the goal of medical education has been and to a large extent still is, to produce healer/scientists. I came out of school assuming that this was the role patients would expect me to fill. I would diagnose and treat disease as I had been taught to do. It never crossed my mind that this would not automatically satisfy patient needs because this is what a doctor is supposed to do. But as soon as I started in practice, I found patients were asking me questions and coming to me with problems that I had no idea how to deal with. Nothing in my schooling had prepared me to deal with them.

The clouded dilemma which emerges is how to improve doctor-patient communication. What is clear, however, is that health professionals and health educators must turn their energies toward developing ways to help physicians meet more of patient needs and to educate the laity to seek to have their needs met in ways which are reasonable, feasible and non-threatening to the provider. Part of the answer to this problem will reside in society's reinforcement of a more equitable relationship between a doctor and patient and a clearer focus of the basic assumptions which underlie joint participation in decision making.

Models of Physician-Patient Interaction

A number of concepts from transactional analysis will be proposed as a working model to clarify the nuances of the physician-patient relationship, and the impact of this interaction on patient responses. This theoretical scheme was selected because the language of transactional analysis is primarily descriptive and educative, rather than exploratory or obtuse [5]. In addition, the key concepts of this theory allow for pragmatic descriptions of different types of universal human interactions and transfer well to the circumstances of doctor-patient relationships. An important factor to bear in mind is that, in any human transaction, two critical components must be addressed: the ways in which the members of the transaction distribute power and control. The struggle around these two issues: who is to initiate and who is to follow, as well as who holds the balance of power in decision making, will determine both the climate of the interaction and the degree of satisfaction derived from it. Therefore, determination of the amount of patient participation which is acceptable in any given doctor-patient interaction should be clarified early in the relationship so that each person has a clear understanding of the responsibilities and expectations of the other.

No one method of doctor-patient interaction is correct for all types of situations. Various models of patient involvement must be tailored to the needs and personality traits of the physician and to the demands of the physical environment in which the service is provided. Information is a precursor to control and a sense of security.

The basic tenet proposed here is not that one model of transaction in medical care is superior to the others, but that certain types work better than others in certain settings. In addition, it is important to recognize that psychological factors (including shared responsibility) may actually play a role in reports of satisfaction with care, as well as have possible impact on the progression or regression of disease. Active participation in decision making and assuming responsibility for one's own treatment has been indicated as a major contributing factor in control of disease and impact on recovery [6]. Feeling helpless and uninvolved in events which affect one's self can be a precursor to feelings of hopelessness and depression, factors often associated with a cancer diagnosis [7]. Individuals who passively accept their disease and adopt a submissive resignation may develop a sense of futility which may progress into a state of dysphoric disillusionment, disinterest in recovery and ultimately a disinclination to live. Recent findings in the literature suggest that angry, active and emotionally expressive patients may actually survive longer [8]. Encouraging a feeling of involvement and giving the patient some sense of control over what is about to take place often elevates mood states, improves psychological adjustment and contributes to a sense of autonomy and self-respect. Therefore, if it is recognized that emotional factors have a significant impact on disease, it would seem reasonable to expect more support from the professional community for the notion that active involvement by patients may have a therapeutic influence. Such an assumption would also carry with it a requirement to discourage patients from suppressing negative feelings and adopting an attitude of stoic acceptance, "no matter how bitter the pill." Understanding that there is a complicated interaction between psychological, transactional and motivational factors in health care is as necessary to providing comprehensive care as are accumulating the necessary medical facts and exhibiting technical expertise.

The following is a brief discussion of three models of physician-patient interaction, all of which have advantages and disadvantages, depending on the circumstances or conditions under which the treatment is to take place [9].

1. *Activity-Passivity*. In this model, the atmosphere is one in which the physician is active and the patient is passive. It is derived from, and is still appropriate for, emergencies, trauma or surgery. The required treatments take place with or without the patient's conscious compliance. The doctor does something to the patient and the patient is regarded as helpless and dependent. Such transaction could be characterized by the "I'm O.K., You're O.K." scheme of transactional analysis in which the physician/parent acts on the patient/child in his/her own best interest, but not necessarily with his/her consent and approval.

2. *Guidance-Cooperation*. This orientation is likely to exist in health care situations that are not so critical or demanding and thus allow a number of alternatives to be considered. A practical illustration might be when a doctor recommends that a patient with terrible back pain and a history of disc problems come into the hospital for traction. Another example may be seen when a physician listens to a patient's chest and says to her that she really should give up smoking because her lungs sound so congested. In both these types of interaction the patient is an adult, alert and responsive, and capable of exercising rational judgment. While this type of transaction allows for some dialogue between participants and the opportunity for the patient to demonstrate intelligent choice, the physician is still viewed as the ultimate authority and judge who pronounces both verdict and sentence. The result often is that the patient initially resists the recommendation, may confront the doctor with all types of rationalizations to refute his argument, but ultimately complies with the request (but not as a result of blind obedience). This type of doctor-patient relationship may be characterized by a model of communication similar to that

which exists between a parent and an adolescent child when there is respect for the young person's view, but ultimate judgment resides with the authority figure who "knows what is best."

3. *Mutual Participation or Shared Responsibility*. This type of physician-patient interaction is the model that is gaining popularity lately, especially among social activists, members of humanistic movements and advocates of patient rights. Patients are becoming more vocal about the desire for a mutual endeavor between two parties who are dedicated to the effective management of a health problem. Such an orientation requires that the physician and patient together view the transaction as a covenant between them which is based on mutual respect, shared dialogue and collaborative endeavors to bring about an improved medical condition. Such a parity of efforts and reciprocity of respect reinforce positive feelings about the quality of medical care being given and enhance the patient's sense of autonomy and self-respect. This model allows for a high level of patient activity but still emphasizes a high regard for the physician's skills, opinions and technical expertise. According to this type of interaction, the physician helps the patient to help herself. In the parlance of transactional analysis, this behavior is characterized by an adult-to-adult communication, with one member having specialized knowledge which the other voluntarily requests and evaluates as to its usefulness. A lucid illustration of this type of transaction would be the case when a physician discusses the risks-benefits of recommending chemotherapy to a breast cancer patient who has one positive axillary node. The patient must be informed about the risks to her body of no treatment of this type, the side effects from this toxic element, and the anticipated benefit of extending her survival by a certain percentage because of the chemical's possible therapeutic effect. The final decision for this treatment should be made after serious deliberation regarding the risks and benefits outlined by the doctor, and after serious consideration on the part of the patient about her own alleged assets vs. disadvantages in taking the treatment. Reactions to such requests are not totally rational and not necessarily a direct outcome of the statistics presented by the doctor to the patient. It is important to remember that the ultimate choice is influenced by a multiplicity of factors. "The patient does not

have the luxury of the physician's distance. The cancer is within her, and more important, treatments the physician prescribes are within her" [9]. Therefore, the final decision should come from within her.

Philosophical Considerations:
The Need for Communication Skills

Parity in decision making and the concept of shared responsibility in medical care are not appropriate for all patients. Individuals of very low intelligence or those who are emotionally unstable may not have adequate skills or impulse control to make rational decisions. Therefore, they may be considered exceptions to this model. The active-participation concept can be used; however, it has not been used as frequently as it might be and resistance to encouraging patients to ask questions or request explanations about their care is still quite prevalent. Education for laity and professionals is necessary to promote more practice of joint participation in decision making and more acceptance of the positive attributes of this level of shared responsibility. "Recognizing and satisfying patients needs — as patients see them — is a major challenge facing physicians in the 1980's. Where the patient was once almost entirely without power, he/she is emerging as a strong influence (which will) shape the quality and direction of medical care. The physician who fails to recognize and respond to this phenomenon does so at his peril" [4].

While this author agrees that the trend in the purchase of medical services seems to be shifting from a seller's to a buyer's market, the most desired change in attitudes will be brought about through enlightenment, not coercion. Therefore it seems prudent to make a recommendation to start with some changes in professional schools' educational programs, e.g. inclusion of courses which focus on communication skills, in addition to providing information about medical technology. As one doctor so aptly described the current state of affairs regarding physician-patient interaction, ". . . the father image of the doctor has been supplanted by the skilled technician whose head is far more important than his heart. The trouble is that the patient misses his heart" [10]. What used to be referred to as "bedside manner" is really a composite of caring, interest and time devoted to dialogue with a needy patient. The time allotment today for verbal discourse is even more curtailed than previously because of the multitude of responsibilities held by the primary physician. In addition, the doctor often lacks clues for recognizing patient needs, which may be camouflaged under a cloak of aggressive bravado or pressured inquiry. People who are often very outspoken and/or ostensibly challenging in their style of interaction are really asking for support and validation of their needs to be heard and understood. Recognizing these behaviors as expressive of underlying distress may make interacting with the "difficult" patient more tolerable and minimize the irritation he/she often elicits.

Patients as Active Participants

Joint participation in medical care decision making is predicated on a belief that the patient has an accurate knowledge base, has been able to assimilate the relevant information, and is motivated to be responsible for his/her health care. This premise therefore requires that patients be taught informed consumer behavior in order to (1) evaluate the accuracy and objectivity of reports of medical issues (e.g. Laetrile, the use of marijuana as an antiemetic), as well as (2) assess and judge the adequacy of physician communication and quality of medical care. The first issue regarding critical evaluation of lay coverage of medical information requires that the patient population acquire reliable guidelines regarding the validity and objectivity of discussion of medical facts. Reporters of medical findings as well as producers of mass media programs dealing with health issues are aware of the potential for personal involvement and emotional reactions that such news elicits. Results are therefore frequently reported in a manner that is somewhat irresponsibile and/or sensational, instead of factual and nonevaluative. Articles filled with unbalanced or highly subjective information can result in the laity's experiencing heightened anxiety, distrust of the mainstream of health care and suspiciousness about the people who provide these services.

Such pressing emotions often provoke panicked efforts to find a solution to a problem which is directed by a compelling urge to *do* something, rather than to take time to make a carefully considered choice based on a full discussion of appropriate alternatives. Patients need to learn that a short delay between diagnosis and definitive treatment is a useful period to think through consequences of certain treatments and to make plans to minimize related morbidity.

The second matter, that of judging the quality of medical service and communication from health professionals, is a highly complex issue. One way to approach an analysis of this problem is to focus on the exchange of information between a physician and patient. This involves an effort to determine how much the patient really wants to learn, how comfortable the physician is in assessing that level of inquiry, as well as how willing he/she is to gratify the individual's need to be told what plans are projected. Critical questions to be explored regarding this issue are the following:

1. What is the patient really asking (i.e. specific facts or reassuring comments)?
2. What kind of information will serve what purpose?
3. When is the appropriate time to introduce such information (e.g. several weeks preoperatively, the night before surgery)?
4. Whose responsibility is it to give specific types of information (e.g. rehabilitation, sex-related information)?
5. How should such information be made available (e.g. printed material, audio slide tapes)?
6. How should the impact of information on the patient's psychological adaptation and decision making be evaluated?

Another issue pertinent to patient participation and physician disclosure is what one hopes to achieve by the information to be communicated. Does the doctor want the patient to understand the risks-benefits of a certain procedure, the range of alternatives which currently exist (and are mandated to be described), or the grave implications related to refusal of a certain therapy? The Royal College of Practitioners put forward a list of questions that each physician should ask himself regarding the purpose of his/her communication. These include: "What must I tell this patient? How much of what I learned about him should he know? What words shall I use to convey this information? How much of what I propose to tell him will

he understand? How will he react? How much of my advice will
he take? What degree of pressure am I entitled to apply?" [10].
Each physician must decide which of the above will be
considered and how a decision will be implemented. Irrespective
of the intent of the communication or the intellectual capacity
of the recipient, one must remember that information regarding
medical care should never be overwhelming in amount or
intensity. Patients should be given only as much information as
they are intellectually able to comprehend, emotionally able to
integrate and capable of acting upon to make some difference in
their medical condition or reaction. What this means is that
suggestions to patients ought to deal with issues or problems the
patient is likely to encounter for which he/she will seek a
solution. Often the most useful type of information is aimed at
helping a patient do something specific about his/her condition
(e.g. call the doctor if heat or discharge persists in the incisional
area). One should not give a description of a possible consequence or anticipated problem without suggesting a remedy
(e.g. "your incision may fill up with fluid, or you may notice an
offensive odor in the area"). Very general, abstract or complex
explanations often confuse patients and leave them with a sense
of fear and helplessness. Such feelings may be a precursor to
anxiety or depression which may produce severe emotional
distress or persistent verbal inquiries to try to allay the
apprehension. Unfortunately, such defensive demandingness is
regarded as irritating by the physician and may shut off his
communication.

Another useful rule of thumb is to try to determine which
patients want maximum information about their illness or
treatment choices and which patients would prefer to know as
little as possible, leaving the responsibility of decision making
and worry up to the doctor. Such distinctions are often difficult
to decipher objectively. Nevertheless, there are some fairly
pragmatic clues which illustrate these differences.

Information Seekers (Monitors) vs. Information
Avoiders (Blunters)

Every doctor has an intuitive method for determining who
wants information and who does not. For example, if a woman
comes into the office for a breast biopsy with a pad, pencil,

small tape recorder and a copy of Rose Kushner's book, "Why Me" [11], one can feel fairly confident that this lady is what is termed a "monitor," or information seeker. If, on the other hand, the patient acts somewhat meek or even stoic, or appears uninformed and does not seem to want to know every much, she is likely to be classified as a "blunter," or information avoider. This type of person would rather be distracted from the full impact of the information with which she is presented. She is the type of person who would most likely choose to listen to Muzac rather than read material describing the etiology of her disease, current treatment options, and/or ethical and legal implications of informed consent. Her response to her physician might be, "You are my doctor and know what is best for me; so I will do whatever you suggest." She is not likely to request a second opinion and would rather have fewer options to evaluate than to work on the task of deciding between several alternatives (of apparently equal end results). The monitor, on the other hand, wants to read all relevant material in all kinds of contexts (medical, lay, popular, news, etc). She will often have a prepared list of questions and an already detailed description of the course of events and possible alternatives she would prefer. She seems almost desperate to know about the events which are about to occur so that she can try to anticipate all likely circumstances. Physicians often experience these types of patients as difficult and/or demanding, but may be less irritated if they understand the underlying needs which drive this behavior. Frequently these patients feel they are not in control and the degree of threat experienced correlates with lack of information.

A recent research project by Miller et al [12], investigating which patients benefit from "high-level" information before a painful gynecological procedure, disclosed a number of findings with significant implications for doctor-patient interaction. In addition, the results of this study tend to clarify what have, until now, appeared to be conflicting findings regarding patients' cognitive styles as they relate to obtaining information about medical care. What the Miller report revealed was that individuals do better when the intensity of information they receive is consistent with their particular coping strategy. For monitors, presentation of voluminous information reduced pain during the actual examination, reduced psychological arousal and reduced hostility immediately following the medical procedure. This group, however, did show signs of increased anxiety before and after the examination. Nevertheless, highly informed monitors said they were more satisfied with the preparation they received even though they reported more distress before and after the actual procedure. Monitors who were given low levels of information relevant to their examination stated that they wanted to know more and were less than satisfied with what they had been told. Blunters (information avoiders) showed the greatest benefit when they did not get extensive information ahead of time. Because low-level information or arousal is congruent with their major coping modalities, too much information may be experienced as overload and felt to be threatening or disorganizing. For this group of patients, minimal information reduces anxiety, depression and fear, as well as limits their psycho-physiological symptoms before and after the examination. In summary, one may assume that the doctor who has a desire to impart lots of medical facts and statistics about treatments and outcome ought to confine such communications to monitors. Minimal disclosure is appropriate for blunters, who should be allowed to pale the impact of threat-relevant information by whatever defensive maneuvers they have available to work with.

While these results are quite preliminary and suspect of generalization to other types of threatening medical procedures, the relationship between level of information disseminated and reports of patient satisfaction or comfort is an impressive subject for continued examination. The relative therapeutic outcome of high or low information is dependent upon the individual patient's coping style and will bear directly on his/her reports of satisfaction with the involved physician. Monitors want lots of information in order to feel satisfied with the quality of care they receive and to lessen the anxiety they experience when their future seems highly unpredictable. However, they will also show evidence of increased physiological distress, but apparently this discomfort is a trade-off for the sensation of security they experience when they are informed about what will transpire. Blunters, on the other hand, generally report a lower level of bodily symptoms but a higher level of satisfaction with the information given, especially if they receive only minimal stimulation. If information is withheld from monitors (even though they feel more subjective distress as a result of learning it), they will report being less satisfied with the quality of interaction with their physician. This last factor may have to do with some internalized process regarding one's sense of being in control and having some notion of what to anticipate regarding proposed medical treatment.

It is too early to make definitive generalizations about these findings, but one cannot ignore the implications for more effective patient care in trying to determine the individual's need for information, the doctor's ethical and psychological responsibility in providing that information, and the best way to mesh these two components.

Prescriptions for Verbal Communication

Another important consideration in the area of verbal communication is that certain principles facilitate good communication, while others obstruct or impede it. In fact, certain types of provider response may actually be intimidating or destructive to the doctor-patient relationship. Because the specific transaction between doctor and patient needs to be individualized and responsive to certain inherent cues (is patient a monitor or blunter, passive or assertive, open or withholding?), no simple recommendation will suffice. However, certain guiding principles can be identified which may be viewed as prescriptions for communication [10]:

1. The purpose (of information) is to effect a change in the recipient's knowledge, attitude and, eventually, his behavior (without increasing his/her anxiety to the point of disorganization).
2. The value is to be judged by its effect on the recipient.
3. Good communication is difficult and must be matched to the knowledge, social background, interests, purposes and needs of the recipient.
4. Communication is effected by words, attitudes, expressions and gestures. (Patients may interpret the lack of eye contact as a basis for deception.)
5. If communication is to change behavior, the required

change in the recipient must be seen by him (her) to have more advantages than drawbacks.

6. To ensure success, feedback is needed. (Patients who do not receive feedback often feel rejected.)
7. Communication demands effort, thought, time and often money.

At some time in the future, physicians will look back at our paucity of communication skills with as much incredulity as we regard our predecessors' use of surgery without anesthesia.

Recommended guidelines for effective communication are intended to help influence physician-patient interaction and not dictate physician style. The above recommendations are also a request to have the doctor personalize the communication and take into account each individual patient's psychological dynamics, need to be a participant in her medical treatments, as well as the specific interpretation she has given to the organ in which she contracted the disease.

Out of this entire array of issues surrounding physician-patient communication, one can distill three dominant themes:

1. What to tell the patient (how much).
2. When to tell the patient.
3. How to tell the patient.

No simple solution exists for these problems, but an overriding principle seems worthy of mention: it is not necessary to tell the patient the whole truth, but the whole of what you tell must be the truth.

Proscriptions for Verbal Communication

The foregoing discussion may be viewed as having put forward some psychosocial prescriptions for communications in medical care. It would be imprudent after such a list of "do's" to exclude a brief discussion of the "don'ts." Therefore attention is called to a few of the proscriptions which are important in talking with patients. The most crucial one for the physician to remember is *never* to be falsely reassuring, especially when there are insufficient data upon which to base a definitive statement. For example, it is destructive to a trust relationship between a woman and her doctor, to have him assure her that her condition is absolutely benign. If such a "guesstimate" (particularly regarding a frozen section) turns out to be false, the woman feels lied to, betrayed, helpless and suspicious of future patient-doctor exchanges. Patients seem to do better tolerating a short period of uncertainty about an impending diagnosis rather than being given a diagnosis, with its attendant emotional sequelae, that gets reversed the next day. Maintaining optimism cannot be achieved by offering absolute guarantees, a condition which cannot be maintained in reality.

Some other recommended proscriptions for doctor-patient communication include requests that the doctor *not be* condescending, ingenuine, inappropriately humorous, overly sympathetic or too rushed to hear what the patient is asking. Certain communication skills and physician reactions can have a double-edged impact: they can be used either to safeguard or to threaten a good working relationship with one's patient. The old model of unilateral decision making implemented by the doctor may actually have infantilized patterns and elicit feelings of victimization, dependency and helplessness — all of which contribute to depression, listlessness and noncompliance. On the other hand, a climate of mutual respect, emanating from a model of shared responsibility, may invite a cooperative alliance which can stimulate patient motivation and participation — two conditions which may possibly influence psychological adaptation and/or physical recovery.

Unfortunately, until very recently no one has paid much attention to the human equation in medical care or to the potential therapeutic or destructive influence which the physician-patient interaction may possess. Medical schools are just now beginning to recognize the implications of communication skills in health care, and the fact that they have been negligent in offering curriculum material to deal with this issue. No other area in the preparation of the trained physician has received so little necessary attention, except that of the role of human sexuality in patient care. Health professionals from all disciplines, but especially medical doctors, are seriously undertrained in effective communication skills and the psychodynamics of the doctor-patient interaction. The old adage that communication is a natural act and one which does not have to be learned does not take into account the fact that the art of communication can be, and often is, improved by specialized training. Given that a new era is emerging in medical care and the unilateral directive of the parental physician is dimming, the education of doctors will have to change to accommodate the new philosophy. Course content which describes the value of patient activism and supports the need for a core list of effective communication skills must be incorporated into the training of our future doctors. Attempts to establish such enlightened attitudes mean encouraging health professionals to respect patient independence as a therapeutic objective and to strive for conditions that will reinforce this goal. Such alterations in our belief system about medical transactions will carry the assumption that the patient and physician are partners in an open-ended health planning contract. There will be fewer and fewer closed-ended arrangements in which the physician is a dictator and the patient passively waits to be directed.

Difficulties between physician and patient in the area of communication interfere with the ability to obtain from the doctor information which is necessary for a truly informed consent, as well as to provide information the doctor may need to make a definitive diagnosis (e.g. occasional bloody discharge from one's nipple). A lack of honest dialogue tends to shut down information offered by the patient which may be useful to the doctor. Barriers in the communication process create obstacles to both upward and downward (or preferably "cross-party") flow of information. Placed in a position of inequity or uncertainty about their "rights," patients may withhold essential information from their doctors because (1) they do not want to bother them, (2) they cannot evaluate the importance of a specific condition or bodily symptom, or (3) they want to manipulate the physician's assessment of their condition for either interpersonal or economic gain. On the other hand, if the patient is open and expressive of her needs, the physician is forced to acknowledge the patient's demand for recognition in the relationship and to deal with it in one of two ways. The doctor may (1) accept the invitation and react to the patient as an adult who is entitled to explanations and answers, or (2) discourage the patient's attempts at participation by employing various communication-limiting strategies. If a patient does not attempt to ask questions during an initial visit, an inequitable pattern is established and the physician assumes dominance in the interaction by default of the patient. Patient ignorance or reticence creates a hothouse for provider power, and patients' fantasies that doctors are larger than life-size contribute to their passivity and timidity.

As mentioned earlier, there is a direct relation between the extent of information received from their physicians and the patients' reports of satisfaction with their health care. In addition, the perception of the physician as friendly, understanding of patient concerns and possessing good communication skills was consistently associated with increased satisfaction and compliance (appointment keeping and following through with instructions for care). Adherence or compliance seems to relate very positively to certain personality characteristics and the level of participation evident in the doctor-patient interaction. Noncompliance, on the other hand, is related to attempts by the physician to control the patient and such other factors as the physician's outright expression of disagreement with the patient, a rejecting or very formal attitude, and a climate of no feedback offered after the doctor has extracted information from the patient. "It appears that, when patients are involved in the decision-making process, they are more likely to accept the responsibilities imposed by their condition and go along with the necessary treatment" [1].

Guidelines for Physician-Patient Communication

The following list of recommendations is an effort to delineate the responsibilities of both parties in establishing a cooperative alliance dedicated to optimum health care and patient satisfaction. These recommended behaviors are predicated on a belief system that values shared responsibility as the prototype of transactions between doctor and patient and, further, affirms a cooperative alliance as the most desirable balance of power in decisions about treatment. Specific guidelines to achieve this goal are listed below.

Patient Responsibilities:

1. To ask for information about treatments, side effects, alternatives.
2. To ask the physician about his training, certification and opinions about "standard" as well as alternative treatments.

3. To let the doctor know if one feels rushed, confused or intimidated.
4. To provide information about one's medical and psychological condition so the doctor can make an accurate assessment of one's condition or illness.
5. To read and question informed-consent contracts and to ask for clarification of terms or outcomes not understood.
6. To ask about fees and arrangements for deferred payment if that is necessary.

Physician Responsibilities:

1. To encourage question asking.
2. To provide relevant information in language and manner the patient can comprehend by determining the patient's need for information (viz. seeker vs. avoider).
3. To provide supplemental written or visual aids to clarify diagnosis and/or treatment.
4. To regard the psychological needs of the patient as an integral part of medical care.
5. To employ strategies which encourage patient adherence to treatment requirements (e.g. written instructions and return postcard for follow-up care).
6. To provide risk-benefit information about standard treatment as well as alternative modes of therapy.
7. To outline and suggest baseline evaluation tests as well as a follow-up program for continued care.

Conclusion

The essence of a mutually cooperative endeavor in health care assumes that reactions from both parties affect the nature and outcome of the interaction. The stimuli from the provider to patient and from patient to provider determine the amount of information that gets disseminated. The type and amount of information and the communication style of the provider have distinct implications for the level of dissatisfaction or gratification experienced by the patient. Therefore it is mandatory to examine the reciprocal flow of factors which shape the doctor-patient transaction. While public testimony is replete with the conviction that physician communications are limited or altered in an attempt to protect patients from emotional upset or worry, a literature review demonstrates conclusions to the contrary. A study by Hershey and Bushkoff revealed that disclosure to patients did not cause them to withhold consent for the recommended treatment [12]. Therefore claims about safeguarding information to protect patients need to be carefully evaluated. What remains to be documented is whether the tide of consumerism in medicine can wash in a new mood, one that is less dictatorial, less paternalistic and more satisfying than that which currently exists. It may be helpful to think of health care not just as an implicit contract to secure services and treatments, but as a special partnership and collaborative endeavor with benefits to be accrued to both participants.

Modern women are moving out of their submissiveness and ignorance regarding the purchase of medical care. They are exhibiting a high level of knowledge, competence and responsibility for their health. They are, in addition, actively demanding a more participatory role in the decisions about the treatments for their disease as well as conditions which influence the quality of their survival. Increased physician-patient partnership can result in improved patient satisfaction, increased adherence to treatment regimens, reduced burdens for the doctor and enhanced feelings of individuality, autonomy and self-respect.

References

1. Kalisch, B.J.: Of half gods and mortals: Aesculapian authority. Nursing Outlook 23 (1):24, 27, 1975.
2. Schain, W.S.: Patients rights in decision making: The case for personalism versus paternalism in health care. Cancer (Suppl.), Aug. 1980.
3. Roter, D.L.: Patient participation in the patient-provider interaction: The effects of patient question asking on the quality of interaction, satisfaction, and compliance. Health Educ. Monogr. Winter 1977, pp. 281-297.
4. Dr. Everyman challenges understanding and meeting patients needs. Patient Care, April 15, 1980, pp. 166, 175, 177.
5. Harris, T.A.: I'm O.K., You're O.K.: A Practical Guide to Transactional Analysis. New York:Harper & Row, 1969.
6. Simonton, O.C., Mathews-Simonton, S. and Creighton, J.: Getting Well Again: A Step-by-Step Self Help Guide to Overcoming Cancer for Patients and Their Families. New York:St. Martin's Press, 1978.
7. Weisman, A.: Early diagnosis of vulnerability in cancer patients. Am. J. Med. Sci. 271 (2):187-196, 1976.

8. Derogatis, L.R., Abeloff, M.D. and Melisaratos, N.: Psychological coping mechanisms and survival time in metastatic breast cancer. JAMA 242 (14):1504-1508, 1979.
9. Hollender, M.H.: The Psychology of Medical Practice. Philadelphia:W. B. Saunders Co., 1958, pp. 6-7.
10. Tonkin, M.E.L.: The lack of communication between doctors and patients. South Afr. Med. J., Oct. 8, 1977, pp. 657, 660.
11. Kushner, R.: Why Me: What Every Woman Should Know About Breast Cancer to Save Her Life. New York:Signet, 1975.
12. Miller, S., Mangan, C.E. and Greed, E.: Which Patients Benefit from Information Before a Gynecological Procedure? When The Doctor Should Tell All. Supported by U.S. NIMH Grant MH 19604-07 and NIH Grant RR-99069, 1978.

Self-Evaluation Quiz

1. Aescalapian authority in medical care refers to what kind of decision making?
   a) Egalitarian
   b) Paternalistic
   c) Irrational
   d) Unilateral
2. The shift in emphasis today in medical care concerns is toward more:
   a) Holistic practice
   b) Active patient participation
   c) Shared responsibility
   d) None of the above
3. The basic social science model referred to in this article is:
   a) Behavioral
   b) Transactional
   c) Psychoanalytic
   d) Gestalt
4. Shared responsibility in decision making most closely resembles what level of transaction:
   a) Parent-child
   b) Child-child
   c) Adult-adult
   d) All of the above
5. Patient compliance is positively correlated with:
   a) Physician concern
   b) Physician dictate

  c) Physician experience
  d) Physician training
6. Which of the following emotions is not necessarily correlated with depression?
  a) Control
  b) Helplessness
  c) Hopelessness
  d) Inadequacy
7. Conditions which minimize depression are:
  a) Recreation
  b) Spontaneity
  c) Control
  d) Joyful surroundings
8. Patients who want to receive maximum information about
   their condition are called:
  a) Blunters
  b) Pragmatists
  c) Coders
  d) Monitors

9. Medical consumerism makes up what percentage of the
   gross national product?
  a) 12%
  b) 24%
  c) 9%
  d) 18%
10. Physician communication should be _____ with
    patients' need to know.
  a) Dissonant
  b) Esoteric
  c) Congruent
  d) Relevant

Answers on page 335.

Breast Cancer —
Posttreatment Considerations

Estrogen Receptor in Primary Breast Cancer

C. K. Osborne, M.D., E. Fisher, M.D., C. Redmond, Ph.D.,
W. A. Knight, M.D., M. G. Yochmowitz, M.D.
and W. L. McGuire, M.D.

Objectives

1. To demonstrate that the estrogen receptor content of a primary breast cancer correlates with the degree of tumor differentiation.
2. To update our original study implicating estrogen receptor as an important prognostic variable in patients with primary breast cancer.
3. To discuss the implications of the estrogen receptor assay in planning treatment for patients with primary breast cancer.

Introduction

A major advance in the treatment of human breast cancer has been the development of the estrogen receptor (ER) assay to predict tumor endocrine dependence. It had been known for many years that about one third of human breast cancers would temporarily regress with an appropriate alteration in the hormonal milieu [1]. However, selection of patients likely to respond to these maneuvers was not very successful [2], and many patients were subjected to the risks of ablative endocrine therapy when the treatment was not likely to be beneficial. The development of another effective approach to the treatment of women with advanced breast cancer, cytotoxic chemotherapy,

C. K. Osborne, M.D., W. A. Knight, M.D., M. G. Yochmowitz, M.D. and W. L. McGuire, M.D., Department of Medicine, University of Texas Health Science Center, San Antonio; and E. Fisher, M.D. and C. Redmond, Ph.D., Department of Pathology, Shadyside Hospital, Pittsburgh, Pa.

reinforced the need for an accurate predictive index of hormonal responsiveness in order to individualize therapy. With the discovery that a protein (ER) was necessary for estrogenic activity, investigators asked whether some breast cancers might contain ER, the measurement of which might serve as a marker for hormone dependence. This hypothesis has now been confirmed [3]; patients with ER-negative tumors rarely respond to endocrine therapy, whereas about 60% of patients with ER-positive tumors have an objective response. Patients with tumors containing very high ER concentrations or those also containing progesterone receptor have response rates approaching 80% [4, 5]. Thus, steroid hormone receptor assays have proven very useful in helping clinicians select patients with endocrine-responsive tumors, enabling them to optimize the use of currently available modalities of treatment, as well as providing new areas of investigation.

Recent studies of ER in patients with primary breast cancer undergoing surgery for their disease have revealed another role for the ER assay as a prognostic factor for recurrence and survival. We and others have reported that patients with ER-positive tumors have a lower recurrence rate and better survival than patients with ER-negative tumors [6-13].

These data are not surprising in light of the cell kinetic studies reported by Meyer et al [14, 15] and Silvestrini et al [16], demonstrating that ER-negative tumors have a more rapid proliferative potential. A good correlation was found among several favorable morphological features, the presence of ER and a low thymidine-labeling index, indicating that tumors with a lower proliferative potential are more likely to be endocrine-dependent.

The relationship between ER and prognosis also is not surprising if one accepts the hypothesis that the presence of ER indicates a relative degree of tumor differentiation toward the normal or nonmalignant state, and that well-differentiated tumors generally tend to be more indolent in their clinical behavior. A recent report by Fisher et al [17] suggests that ER does correlate directly with the presence of several morphological features indicative of tumor differentiation. In the present paper we will present results from a group of patients from San Antonio who underwent mastectomy for primary breast cancer, demonstrating that ER may be a biochemical marker for tumor differentiation. Furthermore, we will update and expand our original study showing that ER is an important independent prognostic variable in patients with primary breast cancer.

ER and Breast Cancer Histopathology

Several morphological variables are thought to correlate directly with the degree of tumor differentiation and indirectly with patient prognosis [18]. These include lymphocyte infiltration into the tumor, evidence of tumor necrosis, the degree of elastosis and the degree of nuclear and histologic atypia. In order to determine whether there is a relationship between the presence of ER and morphological evidence of tumor differentiation, we have studied 147 patients undergoing mastectomy for primary breast cancer in whom we had performed an ER assay.* Histopathologic review was performed by one of us (E.F.) without knowledge of the ER result or the patient's clinical history.

The correlation of ER with nuclear and histologic grade is shown in Table 1. Traditionally, low histologic grade and high nuclear grade correspond to the least morphological atypia or

Table 1. Correlation of ER with Nuclear and Histologic Grade

	% ER-Positive	% ER-Negative
Histologic grade*		
1	100	0
2	93	7
3	61	39
Nuclear grade†		
1	50	50
2	90	10
3	100	0

*As grade increases, the degree of morphological differentiation decreases.

†As nuclear grade increases, the degree of nuclear differentiation increases.

*Fisher, E. et al, manuscript submitted for publication.

best differentiation. A striking association between the presence of ER and a high degree of differentiation is evident. Tumors with histologic grade 1 or nuclear grade 3 (best differentiated) always contained the ER protein. In contrast, poorly differentiated tumors (histologic grade 3, nuclear grade 1) were ER-positive in only 50% to 60% of cases. Tumors of intermediate grade had an intermediate rate of ER positivity. The association between well-differentiated tumors, which have a relatively good prognosis [18], and ER complements the data discussed below purporting that ER has prognostic significance.

Tumor necrosis, the degree of elastosis and lymphocyte cell reaction are also related to the degree of tumor differentiation and have prognostic significance [18]. Marked necrosis, marked cell reaction and absent elastica are features of poorly differentiated breast cancers and are associated with the absence of ER (Table 2). In contrast, the absence of necrosis, marked elastica and absent lymphocyte infiltration were nearly always associated with a positive ER status.

The cumulative data correlating ER with the absence or the presence of one or more of five unfavorable morphological characteristics is shown in Table 3. Tumors containing three or more of these variables were frequently ER-negative (70%). In contrast, 79% of tumors with only one or two of the

Table 2. Correlation of ER with Tumor Necrosis, Elastica and Lymphocyte Infiltration

	% ER-Positive	% ER-Negative
Tumor Necrosis		
Absent	88	12
Moderate	66	34
Marked	10	90
Elastica		
Absent	52	48
Moderate	75	25
Marked	92	8
Lymphocyte infiltration		
Absent	94	6
Moderate	69	31
Marked	46	54

Table 3. Correlation of ER with Prognostically
Unfavorable Morphological Characteristics

Characteristics	% ER-Positive	% ER-Negative
0 Unfavorable	98	2
1 or 2 Unfavorable	79	21
3 or More unfavorable	30	70

Unfavorable characteristics include marked lymphocyte infiltration, marked necrosis, no marked elastica, histologic grade 3 and nuclear grade 1.

unfavorable features were ER-positive. A striking correlation was found for tumors displaying none of the five unfavorable characteristics; 98% of these tumors had a positive ER assay. These studies clearly demonstrate that the presence of ER is linked closely to the degree of breast cancer differentiation.

ER and Prognosis

The results of the kinetic studies showing that ER-positive breast cancers have a low thymidine-labeling index and the pathological studies correlating ER with tumor differentiation provide a rationale for the use of ER as a convenient prognostic indicator in patients with primary breast cancer.

Several years ago we determined the ER status in primary breast tumors at the time of mastectomy in patients with clinically localized disease (stages I and II) as an aid in predicting endocrine responsiveness later at the time of recurrence. Analysis of these data revealed that patients with ER-negative cancers had a higher rate of relapse than patients with ER-positive tumors [6]. The recurrence rate for patients with ER-negative tumors was twice that for patients with ER-positive tumors, an observation which appeared to be independent of other prognostic variables such as age, lymph node involvement, or size and location of the primary. These data suggested that ER-positive tumors are more indolent in their growth behavior than ER-negative tumors. However, this initial study is limited by small patient numbers and short patient follow-up, as well as the fact that the patient population was heterogeneous with regard to the administration of postoperative adjuvant chemotherapy or endocrine therapy.

We have recently updated the study, including additional patients (288 total) and excluding all patients who had received any systemic adjuvant therapy. The median follow-up is now 28 months. The general pattern of results is identical to that observed in our initial study; ER-negative patients are recurring at a significantly higher rate than ER-positive patients. The data shown in Table 4 suggest that ER is an independent prognostic variable. Thirty-five percent of all patients with ER-negative tumors have developed recurrent disease, compared to only 18% of patients with ER-positive tumors. More importantly, regardless of menopausal status, the number of positive axillary nodes or location of the primary in the breast, ER-negative patients are experiencing recurrences at a high rate. The differences are impressive when the patients are stratified by the most important prognostic factor, lymph node status. Only 8% of ER-positive, node-negative patients have had recurrences, compared to more than one fourth of the ER-negative group. These data are important when one considers that node-negative patients are usually excluded from adjuvant chemotherapy because of their "good prognosis" with surgery alone. ER-negative patients with positive axillary nodes have a very bad prognosis; 43% of patients in this group with one to three positive nodes and 68% of those with more than three positive nodes have had recurrences within two years.

Table 4. Recurrence by ER Status and Other Potential Prognostic Factors

| Subgroup | Estimated Recurrence at Two Years (%) | |
	ER-Positive	ER-Negative
All patients	18	35
Menopausal status		
Pre	18	35
Post	15	38
Node status		
0	8	26
1-3	16	43
>3	40	68
Tumor location		
Outer	12	32
Inner + central	12	50

Table 5. Patient Survival at 28 Months by ER Status

ER Status	Mortality (%)		
Total	43/288	(15%)	
Positive	25/207	(12%)	P <.004
Negative	18/81	(22%)	

These patients have now been followed long enough to begin to examine the effect of ER status on survival. Actual patient survival at the time of analysis is shown in Table 5. Fifteen percent of the entire group have died. However, significantly more ER-negative patients (22%) have died as compared to ER-positive patients (12%). The survival advantage of patients with ER-positive tumors holds even when the patients are stratified by nodal status (Figs. 1 and 2). As expected, node-negative patients have the best survival and to date only 10% have died. However, more ER-negative patients have died (14% compared to 8%, a difference which has nearly reached statistical significance). The difference becomes more apparent in the node-positive group (Fig. 2); 43% of ER-negative patients have already died, compared to only 19% of the

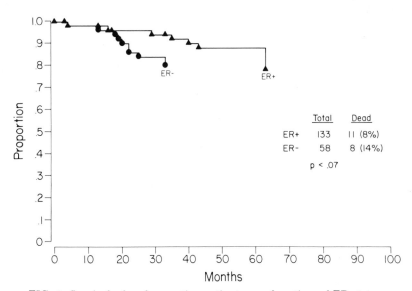

FIG. 1. Survival of node-negative patients as a function of ER status.

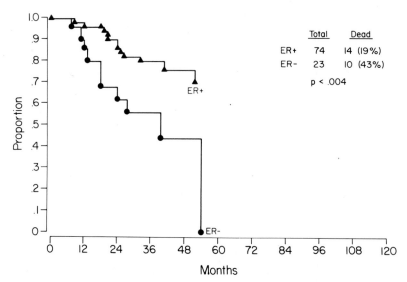

FIG. 2. Survival of node-positive patients as a function of ER status.

ER-positive group. In fact, ER-positive, node-positive patients are dying at a rate very similar to that of ER-negative patients with negative axillary nodes. The prognosis for ER-negative patients is indeed poor.

Thus, these studies indicate that the ER status of a primary breast cancer is an important independent prognostic variable for recurrence and survival of patients with this neoplasm. Several other investigators have now confirmed these results [7-13], but additional follow-up will be required to determine whether these patterns persist with time.

Implications for Therapy of Primary Breast Cancer

The results of these studies, summarized in Table 6, suggest that ER-positive tumors tend to be well differentiated, with a low proliferative capacity which is reflected by their indolent clinical behavior and favorable prognosis. Furthermore, many of these tumors are responsive to endocrine therapy. ER-negative tumors tend to be poorly differentiated, with a high proliferative capacity and aggressive clinical behavior. The risk for recurrence of these tumors is relatively high even when the

Table 6. Summary of ER in Primary Breast Cancer

	ER-Positive	ER-Negative
Degree of differentiation	Good	Poor
Proliferative capacity	Low	High
Clinical behavior	Indolent	Aggressive
Risk of recurrence	Low	High
Endocrine dependence	Common	Rare

axillary nodes are uninvolved with tumors. ER-negative tumors rarely respond to endocrine therapy.

These findings form the framework for a new approach to the treatment of primary breast cancer. It is of obvious importance that clinical studies of new treatments should at least stratify patients by ER status, just as is done for nodal status and other prognostic factors. Moreover, ER may also be used to design new treatment strategies. For instance, axillary node-negative, ER-positive patients have a good prognosis and can probably be managed with local modalities of therapy only. On the other hand, adjuvant chemotherapy (on a research basis only) should be considered in the ER-negative subgroup because of the relatively higher rate of recurrence. Axillary node-positive patients are at a greater risk for recurrence, especially the subgroup with ER-negative tumors. Intensive chemotherapy should be considered for this subgroup in an attempt to control micrometastases and improve the dismal survival. ER-positive patients with positive nodes also have a relatively high risk for recurrence, but the endocrine dependence of many of these tumors permits alternative treatment approaches. Endocrine therapy with or without cytotoxic chemotherapy might be studied in these patients, particularly the postmenopausal subgroup in whom adjuvant chemotherapy alone has not been uniformly beneficial. Clinical trials to answer these important questions are now under way.

References

1. Beatson, G.T.: On treatment of inoperable cases of carcinoma of mamma. Suggestions for a new method of treatment with illustrative cases. Lancet 2:104, 1896.

2. Stoll, B.A.: Hormonal Management in Breast Cancer. Philadelphia:J. B. Lippincott, 1969.

3. McGuire, W.L., Carbone, P.P. and Vollmer, E.P.: Estrogen Receptors in Human Breast Cancer. New York:Raven Press, 1975.

4. Osborne, C.K. and McGuire, W.L.: Current use of steroid hormone receptor assays in the treatment of breast cancer. Surg. Clin. North Am. 58:777, 1978.

5. Horwitz, K.B., McGuire, W.L., Pearson, O.H. and Segaloff, A.: Predicting response to endocrine therapy in human breast cancer: A hypothesis. Science 189:726, 1975.

6. Knight, W.A., Livingston, R.B., Gregory, E.J. and McGuire, W.L.: Estrogen receptor is an independent prognostic factor for early recurrence in breast cancer. Cancer Res. 37:4669, 1977.

7. DeSombre, E.R., Greene, G.L. and Jensen, E.V. In McGuire, W.L. (ed.): Hormones, Receptors and Breast Cancer. New York:Raven Press, 1978, pp. 1-14.

8. Rich, M.A., Furmanski, P. and Brooks, S.C.: Prognostic value of estrogen receptor determinations in patients with breast cancer. Cancer Res. 38:4296, 1978.

9. Allegra, J.C., Lippman, M.E., Simon, R. et al: Association between steroid hormone receptor status and disease-free interval in breast cancer. Cancer Treat. Rep. 63:1271, 1979.

10. Maynard, P.V., Blamey, R.W., Elston, C.W. et al: Estrogen receptor assay in primary breast cancer and early recurrence of the disease. Cancer Res. 38:4292, 1978.

11. Bishop, H.M., Elston, C.W., Blamey, R.W. et al: Relationship of oestrogen-receptor status to survival in breast cancer. Lancet 2:283, 1979.

12. Booke, T., Shields, R., George, D. et al: Oestrogen receptors and prognosis in early breast cancer. Lancet 2:995, 1979.

13. Hahnel, R., Woodings, T. and Vivian, A.B.: Prognostic value of estrogen receptors in primary breast cancer. Cancer 44:671, 1979.

14. Meyer, J.S., Bauer, W.C. and Rao, B.R.: Subpopulations of breast carcinoma defined by S-phase fraction, morphology, and estrogen receptor content. Lab. Invest. 39:225, 1978.

15. Meyer, J.S., Rao, B.R., Stevens, S.C. and White, W.L.: Low incidence of estrogen receptor in breast carcinomas with rapid rates of cellular replication. Cancer 40:2290, 1977.

16. Silvestrini, R., Daidone, M.G. and DiFronzo, G.: Relationship between proliferative activity and estrogen receptors in breast cancer. Cancer 44:665, 1979.

17. Fisher, E.R., Redmond, C.K., Lin, H. et al: Correlation of estrogen receptor and pathologic characteristics of invasive breast cancer. Cancer, 1980. (In press.)

18. Fisher, E.R., Gregorio, R.M. and Fisher, B.: The pathology of invasive breast cancer. A syllabus derived from findings of the National Surgical Adjuvant Breast Project (Protocol No. 4). Cancer 36:1, 1975.

Self-Evaluation Quiz

1. The most important variable in predicting the endocrine dependence of a human breast cancer is:
   a) Previous response to hormonal therapy
   b) Menopausal status
   c) Disease-free interval
   d) Estrogen receptor content
   e) Sites of metastatic disease
2. Which of the following is true regarding estrogen receptor-negative tumors?
   a) They have a high thymidine-labeling index
   b) There is a strong correlation with histologic type
   c) They are frequently hormone-responsive
   d) They have a more favorable prognosis
   e) They are usually well differentiated
3. All of the following are characteristics of good breast tumor differentiation, *except*:
   a) Absent tumor necrosis
   b) Marked elastosis
   c) Marked lymphocyte infiltration
   d) Low histologic grade
   e) A relatively favorable prognosis
4. The presence of estrogen receptor correlates with which of the following?
   a) Marked tumor necrosis
   b) Low histologic grade
   c) Marked lymphocyte infiltration
   d) Absent elastica
   e) Medullary carcinoma
5. Estrogen receptor-positive tumors:
   a) Are more aggressive clinically
   b) Are poorly differentiated
   c) Are more common in node-negative patients
   d) Require adjuvant therapy when axillary nodes are negative
   e) Are less aggressive clinically
6. The estrogen receptor assay on a primary breast tumor may help the physician in all but which of the following:
   a) Planning which hormonal therapy is optimal

VANDERBILT MEDICAL CENTER LIBRARY

    b) Selecting high-risk subgroups for adjuvant therapy
    c) Identifying endocrine therapy-responsive tumors
    d) Selecting hormonal therapy or chemotherapy at the time of relapse
    e) Designing new adjuvant treatment approaches

Answers on page 335.

Breast Reconstruction Following Mastectomy for Malignant Disease: A Surgical Oncologist's Point of View

Gordon F. Schwartz, M.D.

Objectives

The purpose of this paper is to acquaint the reader with the current status of breast reconstruction in general terms and to encourage a frank and open discussion of this subject between physicians and patients.

Cancer of the female breast occupies its unique position as one of the most formidable and threatening afflictions of modern times because of the fear engendered by the contemplated treatment, in addition to the usual anxiety and concern for survival which accompanies the diagnosis. Not infrequently, women with breast lumps delay reporting their findings to their physicians, fearing that mastectomy may be the "reward" for their diligence and early detection of breast cancer. This fear of treatment is compounded by the generally fatalistic approach that breast cancer is uniformly progressive and invariably lethal, so why bother?

Psychiatrists and psychologists have little difficulty recognizing that the fear of treatment may play a significant role in delayed diagnosis, since, to some women, the cure is worse than the disease. We must attempt to educate women that early

Gordon F. Schwartz, M.D., F.A.C.S., Professor of Surgery, Jefferson Medical College; Director of Clinical Services, Breast Diagnostic Center, Thomas Jefferson University Hospital, Philadelphia, Pa.

Reprinted, with permission, from Clinics in Plastic Surgery, Vol. 6, No. 1, January 1979.

detection of breast cancer leads not only to increased survival, but also that earlier and earlier detection may lead ultimately to the day when breast cancer may be diagnosed at a stage at which removal of the breast is rarely necessary.

Unfortunately, we have not yet reached this goal, and some form of mastectomy — radical or modified radical, occasionally total (simple) mastectomy — is the usual treatment for most forms of breast cancer. These operations, even when skillfully performed, lead to disfigurement that is difficult to accept by many women. Even partial mastectomy or lumpectomy, more often than their proponents are willing to admit, leads to significant distortion of the breast. Whether or not the physical scars may be covered by an external prosthesis, making the patients outwardly no different from other "normal" women, the inner emotional scars remain. The prospect of breast reconstruction, therefore, is a subject of intense contemporary interest, and has received considerable publicity, bordering on notoriety, in the nonmedical press. Techniques of surgery have advanced enough so that the question is not whether reconstruction can be performed, but rather, should it be performed?

The advisability of reconstruction following mastectomy for malignant breast disease evokes heated debate among physicians. As with other medical controversies, there are reputable physicians taking both sides of the argument, each equally convinced that his alone is the proper approach. How can any woman, especially one so psychologically as well as physically traumatized by mastectomy, reach a reasonable conclusion as to the best course to follow? If reconstruction were accepted universally as the final stage of the treatment program for the basic disease, rather than as a unique procedure, available only to certain selected women, perhaps campaigns to achieve earlier detection of breast cancer would be more readily accepted. It seems reasonable to assume that more women would join screening programs, for example, if their diligence and motivation led to more than just the loss of a breast.

Arguments cited that oppose reconstruction include the likelihood of masking recurrent cancer, or of activating dormant cancer cells that may have been present microscopically but had not been biologically active, or of altering some immune status that had been protecting the patient against recurrence. These arguments are not based upon hard data, but only upon a great deal of folklore and mysticism. What is needed is a more open exposition of the state of the art of reconstruction — what it may hope to accomplish, how it is performed, and when it should be considered. Are there specific precautions to be observed when and if it is undertaken?

Of greatest importance, it is incumbent upon all physicians who treat women with breast cancer to initiate a discussion of possible breast reconstruction when the likelihood of mastectomy becomes evident. The exact timing of such a discussion is dictated by the individual patient's circumstances, but the knowledge that reconstruction is possible may help to alleviate significant anxiety well before biopsy and/or mastectomy has been performed. Patients themselves should not bear responsibility for taking the initiative, because even medically sophisticated women may not believe that reconstruction is applicable in their own particular situations. A woman may be too bashful to inquire, embarrassed by what she might believe mistakenly to be only an expression of vanity. Unfortunately, it is all too frequent and incorrect an assumption by a physician that his particular patient would not be interested in reconstruction: "After all, she's over 60," or "She never had a good figure, anyway." One patient we remember best who was most upset by the threatened loss of her breast was in her 80s, not her 20s or 30s. Other surgeons callously feel that women should be satisfied enough just to be rid of their cancers, but fortunately, this group is becoming smaller in number as more physicians hearken to the emotional as well as physical needs of their patients.

There are, undoubtedly, complex psychological reasons why some women, more than others, desire reconstructive surgery following mastectomy, despite the apparent adequacy of their external prosthesis and their appearance when clothed. The best single word coined to describe this complicated interplay of factors is "self-image." Generally, it is those women who were most attentive to their appearance before mastectomy who are most concerned afterward, as might be expected. There are, however, notable exceptions. Many beautiful women who have undergone mastectomy have never bothered with subsequent reconstruction. They are otherwise quite secure, and the loss of one breast has not interfered with their activities, marred their sensuality or, more important, lessened their opinions of themselves.

In this sense, reconstruction of the breast after mastectomy is not unlike other plastic surgical procedures on the breast, i.e. augmentation or reduction mammoplasty. Many of the reasons these operations are sought are buried deeply in the subconscious, and the external appearance of the breast is only one manifestation of the woman's overall ego strengths and weaknesses. As with the other operations, the creation of a new breast may not alter the underlying problem, if there is one; it merely corrects one symptom, albeit a strikingly obvious one!

The physical and emotional turmoil that accompanies the threat of mastectomy is apparent at the inception of the physician-patient dialogue, and an oft-repeated complaint is that women are never fully informed of what is going on, what is planned, and what are the consequences. For example, the need for biopsy and histologic documentation of a lump in the breast may be explained in detail, as well as the possible necessity of some sort of mastectomy. The very mention of the word "cancer," however, even as a remote possibility, is so frequently intimidating that many women recall only bits and snatches of any subsequent discussion. It is most essential that the surgeon reiterate the plans for treatment of her particular problem to each woman, time after time, if need be.

Two particular items of concern are often overlooked during these discussions. The first is the physician's assurance that he is, indeed, aware of the depression, frustration and even anger experienced by the patient when confronted by the diagnosis of cancer. The probable best response by a physician to these emotions is to point them out to the patient as expected and normal, considering the circumstances, then facing them squarely and honestly. Second is the preoperative discussion of the possibilities of reconstruction, should mastectomy be necessary. Elaborate details are unnecessary. Just knowing that such a procedure is remotely possible may help a woman to face the prospect of losing a breast with greater equanimity. It has even been suggested that the more a patient is educated about reconstruction before the need arises, i.e. before mastectomy, the less likely is she to focus on this procedure as a "must" after the mastectomy.

Another valid reason why reconstruction of the breast is an appropriate subject for discussion before acquiescing to mastectomy may be to learn the surgeon's ideas about the placement of the mastectomy incision and the actual technique to be employed. The initial surgical procedure and the manner in which the mastectomy is accomplished often determine how much may be achieved and how difficult a later reconstruction may prove to be. Even if a woman were to choose not to undergo reconstruction, a properly placed incision makes it easier for her to select and wear clothing. For example, there is no need for the surgical incision for mastectomy to cross the shoulder and on out onto the upper arm, or to extend into the hair-bearing portion of the underarm. Most experienced surgical oncologists now use either a transverse incision or a vertical incision in the strap line. At the conclusion of the mastectomy, when the skin flaps are replaced on the chest wall, it is also possible to mold these flaps to recreate as much of the preoperative appearance as possible. It may be impossible to avoid entirely the defect produced by the loss of the pectoralis major muscle if radical mastectomy is necessary, but the axillary hollow may be minimized and made less conspicuous by careful placement of the original incision and molding these skin flaps carefully.

Even radical mastectomy does not doom a patient to a lifetime of high-collared, long-sleeved dresses. With a proper prosthesis and a carefully placed incision, mastectomy patients may wear clinging, sleeveless or scoop-necked dresses without fear that anyone might guess that they had lost one breast. If more surgeons took greater pains to plan their incisions carefully, perhaps there would be fewer women who would demand reconstruction, since the ultimate defect would be lessened.

Regardless of the patient's desire for reconstruction, it must never be forgotten that the operation is being done for a dangerous disease, and insufficient or inadequate treatment may prove fatal. Compromising on the operative procedure demanded by the cancer encountered, just to be able to perform subsequent reconstruction, is "bad" medicine. It is certainly a woman's privilege to choose the surgeon and the operation, or nonoperation, to treat her particular problem, but as conscientious physicians, it is our responsibility to acquaint our patients with both the benefits and the risks of proposed treatment. If a procedure is demanded by a woman, and we do not agree with that particular treatment for that specific problem, it is also our duty to explain the consequences of that mode of therapy, at least as we perceive them. All too often, a woman will shop for a physician who will tell her what she wants to hear, whether or not his advice is appropriate for her particular clinical situation. Dialogue that includes discussion about reconstruction may, in part, remove some of the immediate depression and anxiety that accompany the diagnosis, and also lessen the likelihood of a woman shopping for an opinion more to her liking. Second opinions are not deprecated, so long as the physician chosen to render that opinion is knowledgeable, not merely accommodating or gratuitous.

Thus it is preferable to suggest to the patient about to undergo mastectomy that reconstruction is possible, regardless of the nature of the mastectomy performed. Certainly, some operations and incisions, as noted, lend themselves better to later reconstruction, and when feasible, these should be employed; but the procedure recommended and chosen to treat the cancer must offer the patient the highest chance for survival.

The timing of reconstruction, should one choose to proceed, is also a matter of controversy. There are some surgeons who advocate trying to place some form of implant beneath the skin flaps of the mastectomy wound, just to restore even a portion of the breast mound to the patient immediately. This approach has been suggested to make the patient aware of the better reconstruction yet to come and to minimize her feelings of mutilation. Unfortunately, it is infrequent that an initial implant, even after total mastectomy alone without lymph node dissection, if it has been a proper cancer operation, will be large enough or in the proper position not to require operative replacement or adjustment in the future. We have generally discouraged this approach except in most unusual circumstances.

One reason to postpone reconstruction is the emotionally vulnerable status of any woman at the time of mastectomy. If offered, there are probably few women who would not choose immediate reconstruction, mentally suppressing or ignoring the likelihood of subsequent revisions. Also, many women to whom the prospect of reconstruction appears so attractive initially lose their zeal for it after their wound has healed and they become accustomed to their external prosthesis. The realities of their situation are not so bad as their expectations had led them to believe, as is so often the case when dealing with any formidable and threatening experience.

If, as we generally recommend, reconstruction is deferred until wound healing has been completed, it does mean a delay of at least six months, often longer. Full arm motion should be regained and the patient should resume unrestricted activity before any thought of reconstruction. It is a natural assumption that women who have undergone radical mastectomy, with the loss of both pectoral muscles, take longer to heal than women who have undergone lesser operations, such as modified radical mastectomy, with the pectoralis major muscle spared. This is not necessarily so! When the muscle has been removed in its entirety, healing and recovery of arm motion often occur more rapidly than when the muscle has been retracted forcibly to expose the underlying structures of the axilla, and its fascia has been excised completely, as must be accomplished in an adequate modified radical mastectomy.

Until recently, it had been the admonition of many oncologists that reconstruction should be deferred until one was fairly certain that the patient had little chance of wound recurrence. This argument was accepted by a majority of physicians and patients, until women began to voice their opinions that the quality of life should be equated in importance to the quantity of life. It is unfortunate that not all women are cured of their cancer, regardless of the stage of the disease when detected or the treatment employed. However, if the operation chosen to treat the cancer initially is appropriate to the situation and performed meticulously, even among those women destined to succumb to recurrent cancer, only a very small proportion will ever develop recurrence at the operative site. Withholding reconstruction until cure was a virtual certainty because of the possibility of masking local recurrence may have been a valid argument back in the days when many women undergoing mastectomy had more advanced disease. Present criteria of operability minimize the likelihood of such wound recurrence.

Although the chance of recurrence must be one factor to be weighed when a woman considers the advantages and disadvantages of reconstruction, only she can make the final decision, based upon her own list of priorities. Such a decision must be the patient's prerogative. The physician's duty may be to inform her of the statistical chances of recurrence, but this fact alone should not deter her from contemplating reconstruction. For some women, the high possibility of recurrent disease might be a reason to accelerate reconstruction, so they might be "whole" again, for whatever period of life remains. On the other hand, it would be ill-advised to embark upon a program that might entail several procedures and take more than one year to complete if recurrence were quite likely. There are presumably infinitely better ways to spend that year than running back and forth between doctor's office and hospital.

When reduction of the remaining breast is recommended as part of the overall plan for reconstruction, more heated debate is generated about the propriety of reconstruction. There is no doubt that the remaining breast is at increased risk for the development of cancer in any woman who has already had cancer of one breast. This risk, for women whose first cancer occurred prior to menopause, may be as high as 15 times the normal expectation. Any operative procedure on the remaining breast is therefore viewed as possibly masking the early detection of a contralateral cancer. Some aggressive surgeons have suggested that the remaining breast be removed altogether by subcutaneous mastectomy or total mastectomy, and replaced by an implant, to protect the patient from the chance of this second cancer.

We do not concur with those who advocate either subcutaneous mastectomy or prophylactic total mastectomy. The former procedure may leave behind as much as 20% of the breast tissue, if it is performed to maximize the aesthetic appearance of the breast, and it implies preservation of the nipple-areolar complex. Approximately 30% of breast cancers arise within 1 cm of the areolar margin or 1 cm deep to the nipple and areola; therefore, we do not consider subcutaneous mastectomy to be as good a preventive measure against cancer as often advertised. Total mastectomy, which includes removal of the axillary tail, certainly should prevent cancer, but this is indeed a bitter pill for women to swallow after they have already undergone amputation of the first breast. Instead, we advocate frequent folow-up of any patient with breast cancer, including quarterly clinical examination, and bone scan, SMA-12 and mammogram of the remaining breast at annual intervals. Should a second cancer occur, this type of follow-up has a high likelihood of detecting it at a time when the possibilities of "cure" are highest.

We do not have the same negative opinion about reduction of the contralateral breast as part of the reconstructive procedure, so long as the patient is cautioned about the need for careful follow-up. The reduced breast often demonstrates changes in texture and consistency related to the operative procedure, and every precaution must be taken to ensure that something new developing in that breast is not missed. Again, it is crucial that the patient be informed of these concerns and participate in the final decision.

When reconstruction is anticipated, according to the usual timetable at least six months after the initial operative procedure, it would be prudent to ensure that there is no evidence of recurrence, within the limits of current medical practice. As noted, annual work-up is the rule, including bone scan, SMA-12 and mammogram of the opposite breast, either by film or xeromammography. Selected patients also should undergo liver and/or brain scans and skeletal survey. If the timing of the reconstruction occurs prior to the anniversary of the mastectomy, before the usual annual work-up has been performed, it is best to proceed with these studies before the reconstruction is initiated. If any of these examinations proves suspicious or suggestive of recurrent disease, investigation of the abnormal findings would then take precedence over reconstruction. The procedure should be postponed, not necessarily canceled.

Many women with histologic evidence of axillary node metastases are now enrolled in adjuvant chemotherapy programs for periods of one to two years following mastectomy. Although there are no data that relate wound healing to the administration of adjuvant chemotherapy, it is accepted that these agents exert a deleterious effect on wound healing, at least in the doses used to treat recurrent disease. Although the doses of the drugs used in most of the adjuvant chemotherapy protocols are lower, and the intervals between administration minimize the side effects, it is probably better to postpone consideration of reconstruction for these patients until the adjuvant chemotherapy has been completed. If recurrence has not occurred by that time, reconstruction may then proceed. There is no reason why the patient receiving adjuvant chemotherapy cannot visit with the reconstructive surgeon and make the necessary plans, even if the implementation of these plans is delayed until after the chemotheraphy has been completed.

Finally, many women who might otherwise consider reconstruction of the breast following mastectomy for cancer shy away from discussing this with their physicians because of concerns about cost. Since this procedure is, in one sense, a cosmetic operation, it is often viewed by patients as an indulgence to their vanity. As such, they are often unwilling to commit what might be a large portion of a family budget to so-called elective or unnecssary surgery, especially if their budget has just withstood the onslaught of hospitalization for mastectomy. Fortunately, more and more medical insurance plans have begun to realize that these operations are more than just cosmetic surgery, and are often necessary for the psychological, if not physiological, health of the patient. Even though the very same insurance carriers may not honor the costs of other aesthetic breast surgery, they have demonstrated interest in the overall rehabilitation of the cancer patient by accepting responsibility for at least some of the costs of reconstruction. As more and more physicians, patients and organizations, such as the American Cancer Society, express their opinions and exert their combined influence, we may expect that other insurance carriers will be willing to accept their fiscal responsibilities to their policyholders in this regard.

Thus, there is almost no woman who has undergone mastectomy, regardless of the "radicalness" of the procedure, who is not a candidate for reconstruction. When properly performed, reconstruction does not increase a woman's risk for recurrence. As previously emphasized, the first priority must be the attempted eradication of the cancer by whatever technique is deemed most likely to do so. This initial and most important step having been completed, reconstruction of the breast then becomes a subject of variable priority depending upon the patient's own point of view, as well as the likelihood of recurrent cancer.

Summary

The various factors that enter into the decision and recommendation for breast reconstruction after mastectomy must include the time and number of procedures which may be required and the probability of recurrent cancer, but most of all, the degree of enthusiasm of the woman herself for the procedure. Only a small percentage of women who initially express interest in reconstruction actually carry it through to completion, for many reasons. What may have been considered initially as a "must" may lose its attractiveness with the passage of time and the realization that mutilation need not be an absolute synonym for mastectomy. Since there is no perfect reconstruction yet available, there cannot be any arbitrary and dogmatic rules established to separate the "should's" from the "should not's." We must await more technical advances from innovative surgeons and biomedical scientists before that millenium arrives. Concurrently, we must endeavor to find techniques of earlier and earlier detection, in the ultimate hope that the diagnosis of breast cancer may be made at a time early enough in its natural history that mastectomy would no longer be required and cure would be guaranteed!

Self-Evaluation Quiz

1. Reconstruction of the breast is to be avoided because of the strong likelihood that it may mask recurrent cancer.
   a) True
   b) False
2. Most incisions currently used for mastectomy, whether radical or modified radical, are placed in such a manner as to make breast reconstruction all but impossible.
   a) True
   b) False
3. Reconstruction is best performed at the same time as the mastectomy whenever possible.
   a) True
   b) False

4. Subcutaneous mastectomy as usually performed is a very effective cancer prophylactic procedure because it removes almost the entire volume of breast parenchyma.
   a) True
   b) False
5. About what proportion of mammary carcinomas arise within the area 1 cm contiguous to or deep to the nipple-areolar complex?
   a) 10%
   b) 30%
   c) 50%
   d) 80%

Answers on page 335.

Utilization of Plasma Marker Proteins for Detection and Monitoring Therapy in Metastatic Breast Carcinoma

Darrow E. Haagensen, Jr., M.D., Ph.D., Sheree Ammirata, R.N.,
Edwin Cox, M.D., William G. Dilley, Ph.D.
and Samuel A. Wells, Jr., M.D.

Objective

The purpose of this paper is to present findings of research studies of carcinoembryonic antigen and human breast gross cystic disease fluid protein as biomarkers for detection and monitoring therapy in metastatic breast carcinoma.

Over the past decade medical research has explored the possibility of detecting and monitoring cancer by analyzing blood samples for specific proteins produced by the cancer cells. In breast carcinoma a number of different molecules have been under investigation as candidate biomarkers. These molecules include enzymes (sialyltransferase [1], alkaline phosphatase [2]); internal cell components (ferritin [3]); cell membrane components (T-blood group substance [4], lymphocyte adherence inhibition antigen [5]); placental/fetal expressed substances (carcinoembryonic antigen [6-9], human chorionic gonadotropin [10], human placental lactogen [11], α-fetoprotein [12]); and components of breast cell secretions

Darrow E. Haagensen, Jr., M.D., Ph.D., Mallory Institute of Pathology, Boston, Mass.; Sheree Ammirata, R.N., William G. Dilley, Ph.D. and Samuel A. Wells, Jr., M.D., Department of Surgery; and Edwin Cox, M.D., Department of Medicine, Duke University Medical Center, Durham, N.C.

(K-casein [13], α-lactalbumin [14], human breast gross cystic disease fluid protein [15]).

The two breast carcinoma biomarkers which our research group has studied in detail are carcinoembryonic antigen (CEA) and a human breast gross cystic disease fluid protein of 15,000-dalton monomer molecular size (GCDFP-15). These two glycoproteins are both useful plasma biomarkers for a proportion of patients with disseminated breast carcinoma.

Methods

Carcinoembryonic antigen was first isolated by Gold and Freedman in 1965 [16, 17]. The commercial radioimmunoassay (RIA) for CEA was developed by Hansen [18, 19]. Several research groups have published reports on the clinical use of CEA plasma levels in detecting and monitoring therapy for breast carcinoma [7-9, 12, 20]. Abnormal CEA levels have been defined as being above 2.5 ng/ml to 10 ng/ml [7-9, 20-22]. In any assay the higher the abnormal level is set, the better the specificity becomes (less false-positives), but the poorer the sensitivity (less true-positives). Our research group has utilized a CEA level above 10 ng/ml as being distinctly abnormal [20]. This level was chosen due to an empirical impression that for patients with a significant carcinoma burden, changes in CEA levels below 10 ng/ml could result from biological phenomena other than alteration in disease status with therapy. In contrast, for CEA levels above 10 ng/ml, alterations in serial CEA levels have, in general, closely correlated with changes in disease status.

With the Hansen assay for CEA a transition zone occurs for CEA levels above 20 ng/ml, where the assay procedure requires changing from analysis of perchloric acid-extracted plasma samples to direct analysis of plasma samples [22]. This shift in assay methodology has added significant confusion to serial CEA trends, as pointed out by Kupchik et al [23].

Our research group has modified the Hansen assay for CEA to utilize only perchloric acid-extracted samples prepared by buffer exchange columns [24]. For CEA levels above 20 ng/ml we aliquot a portion of the assay sample into the standard-curve EDTA buffer. By this methodological change the artifactual shift in apparent CEA levels that can occur with indirect vs. direct CEA analysis is avoided.

The gross cystic disease fluid protein radioimmunoassay was developed by Haagensen for a 15,000 monomer-sized component (GCDFP-15) of this human breast fluid [25]. A normal plasma range of 0 to 80 ng/ml (mean value 30 ng/ml) was established by analysis of blood samples from 150 normal women. Analysis of blood from women with gross cystic disease indicated over half had GCDFP-15 plasma levels above 50 ng/ml, and approximately 20% had plasma levels between 100 and 150 ng/ml [15].

A distinctly abnormal plasma level of GCDFP-15 was empirically set as being above 150 ng/ml. In patients with metastatic breast carcinoma, plasma levels of GCDFP-15 have been recorded up to 70,000 ng/ml. All other major forms of malignancy in women (lung, colon-rectum, ovary, uterus, cervix, pancreas, stomach) have not demonstrated any plasma elevations of GCDFP-15 above 150 ng/ml [15, 26, 27].

Results

An evaluation of CEA and GCDFP-15 plasma levels in 164 women with Columbia stage A or B breast carcinoma has been reported [15, 20]. Neither marker protein was present in the plasma of these women at levels chosen as being distinctly abnormal (CEA >10 ng/ml and GCDFP-15 >150 ng/ml). Only 7 (4%) of the 164 patients had CEA levels between 5 and 10 ng/ml. The use of either CEA or GCDFP-15 plasma levels to detect breast carcinoma at the time it is first clinically evident by palpation is thus limited.

Utilization of Plasma Markers
for Detection of Metastatic
Breast Carcinoma

Over the past four years 235 postmastectomy patients have been evaluated in the Breast Oncology Clinic at Duke University Medical Center by routine screening procedures for development of metastasis, as well as by serial plasma level determinations of CEA and GCDFP-15. Fifty-eight of these patients have developed metastatic recurrence of breast carcinoma documented by biopsy, x-ray or radionuclide scan. An average of 10 serial measurements (range 2-29) of CEA and GCDFP-15 plasma levels was obtained on the 58 patients during the "disease-free interval" prior to clinical detection of metastasis.

Depicted in Table 1 are the findings in the 58 patients who have developed metastatic disease. They are stratified for the predominant location of metastasis at the time of clinical detection vs. the number of patients who had developed elevated plasma levels of CEA only, GCDFP-15 only, or both markers. Of the 23 (40%) patients with elevated plasma levels of CEA and/or GCDFP-15 (Tables 2 and 3) 15 (26%) had the initial elevation in marker level occur prior to the clinical diagnosis of metastasis (range 21 to 693 days prior to clinical diagnosis).

Logarithmically increasing abnormal plasma marker levels were observed in 16 patients by the time of clinical recurrence. Once a logarithmically increasing plasma marker profile appeared, it persisted until clinical detection of metastasis and initiation of therapy. In four patients logarithmically increasing plasma marker values were observed during the entire period in which the measurements were made. A patient with this type of profile is depicted in case 1 (Fig. 1):

Case 1. A 64-year-old black female underwent a left modified radical mastectomy and prophylactic right simple mastectomy in May 1975, with a diagnosis of infiltrating ductal carcinoma in the left breast. Eight of 16 left axillary lymph nodes were involved with metastases. No carcinoma was found in the right breast. The patient was started on adjuvant Cytoxan, methotrexate and 5-fluorouracil (CMF) chemotherapy in June 1975, and followed monthly. Her chemotherapy was discontinued in May 1976. Plasma levels of CEA and GCDFP-15 were first obtained in October 1975. The GCDFP-15 became elevated at 150 ng/ml in December 1975, then doubled every two months

Table 1. Postmastectomy Patients at the Time of
Clinical Detection of Metastatic Breast Carcinoma

Metastatic Disease Location	Number of Patients	GCDFP-15 >150 ng/ml Only	CEA >10 ng/ml Only	Both Markers Elevated	Total Markers Elevated
Soft tissue	23	1	2	0	3 (13%)
Osseous	19	5	5	3	13 (68%)
Visceral	16	3	3	1	7 (44%)
Total	58	9 (16%)	10 (17%)	4 (7%)	23 (40%)

Table 2. Postmastectomy Patients with CEA Levels > 10 ng/ml at the Time of Clinical Detection of Metastatic Breast Carcinoma

CEA Level at Detection of Metastasis (ng/ml)	Location of Metastasis	Total Patient DFI* in Days	Observed Days CEA >10 ng/ml During DFI
520	Bone	747	129 (17%)
52	Bone	1813	35 (2%)
52	Bone	299	299 (100%)
45	Bone	1800	315 (17%)
39	Lung	298	91 (31%)
38	Bone	508	468 (92%)
30	Lung	660	70 (11%)
29	Lung	1345	0
27	Bone	1141	49 (4%)
15	Bone	912	0
14	Bone	1167	693 (59%)
12	Lung	716	0
12	Soft	1160	0
10	Soft	1482	0

*Disease-free interval (DFI) = Time in days between surgery and first clinical detection of the presence of metastases.

Table 3. Postmastectomy Patients with GCDFP-15 Levels > 150 ng/ml at the Time of Clinical Detection of Metastatic Breast Carcinoma

GCDFP-15 Level at Detection of Metastasis (ng/ml)	Location of Metastasis	Total Patient DFI in Days	Observed Days GCDFP-15 >150 ng/ml During DFI
6950	Lung	1345	259 (19%)
6500	Lung	537	343 (64%)
1430	Bone	1813	217 (12%)
738	Lung	667	0A*
711	Bone	1141	120 (11%)
673	Bone	315	0A
480	Bone	490	21 (4%)
335	Bone	1800	315 (18%)
330	Bone	865	209 (24%)
210	Bone	797	0
195	Soft	84	84 (100%)
178	Bone	1534	61 (4%)
177	Liver	567	0A

*A = Time interval between serial GCDFP-15 measurements of greater than 180 days.

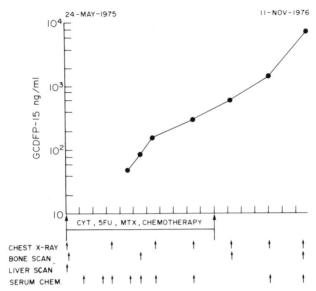

FIG. 1. Plot of the serial GCDFP-15 plasma levels in a postmastectomy patient between the time of surgery and first clinical detection of recurrence. Date at top left is time of surgery. Date at top right is first clinical recurrence. Arrows at bottom indicate when x-ray, scan and serum chemistries were performed. Time axis is marked in 30-day intervals. The CEA level in this patient was consistantly below 4 ng/ml.

to a plasma level of 6500 ng/ml by November 1976, when the patient developed clinical symptoms of left hip pain. Metastasis was documented by bone scan and x-ray of the left pelvis, left femur and chest. The chest x-ray three months earlier (in August 1976) had been normal and the bone scan six months earlier (in May 1976) had been negative. The CEA plasma level was below 4 ng/ml and stable for the entire monitored time interval.

In 12 of the monitored patients there was an initial stable phase of the plasma markers which was followed by serial logarithmically increasing values. In these patients the log-phase elevations preceded clinical detection from one to nine months. A patient with this type of profile is described in case 2 (Fig. 2):

Case 2. A 49-year-old white female underwent a right radical mastectomy in March 1975, with a diagnosis of in

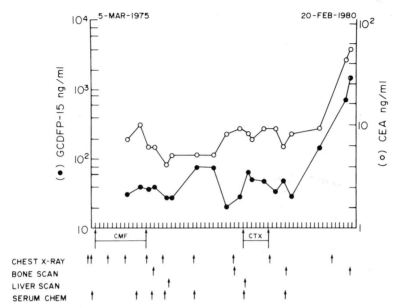

FIG. 2. Plot of serial GCDFP-15 and CEA plasma levels in a postmastectomy patient between the time of surgery and the first clinical detection
of recurrence.

situ and infiltrating lobular carcinoma. Three of three
axillary lymph nodes contained metastases. She was
referred to Duke Medical Center Breast Clinic in April
1975, and was started on combination adjuvant CMF
chemotherapy. Her adjuvant chemotherapy was discontinued in April 1976.

In March 1978, the patient was put on low-dose oral
Cytoxan because her CEA values were still moderately
elevated (4.0 to 9.4 ng/ml). The patient was known to be a
heavy smoker. She was followed monthly and the chemotherapy was discontinued in September 1978. In July
1979, the CEA was at 9.0 ng/ml and the GCDFP-15 had
risen to 142 ng/ml, but there was no evidence of recurrent
disease. In January 1980, a chest x-ray revealed a healing
rib fracture, but a pathological cause could not be
determined; the CEA was 40.7 ng/ml and the GCDFP-15
was 700 ng/ml. In February 1980, a bone scan was positive
for metastases, a biopsy of a right axillary node was

consistent with metastasis, and a bone marrow biopsy also revealed carcinoma cells. The CEA at this time was 52 ng/ml and the GCDFP-15 was 1,430 ng/ml.

The logarithmically increasing plasma marker levels were analyzed for doubling time (Table 4) which varied from 42 to 247 days, with an average of 106 days. The doubling times for the plasma marker levels were similar to the breast carcinoma doubling times which have been determined for serial measurements of tumor size of skin lesions [28] and for increasing size of metastatic lung nodules detected by serial chest x-rays [29].

Table 4. Doubling Time of Logarithmically Increasing
Plasma Marker Protein Levels in 16 Patients
Prior to Clinical Detection of Metastasis

Patient	Observed Log-Phase Doubling Time in Days	P Value	r Value	Abnormal Marker
1.	42	.16	.971	CEA
2.	49	.27	.969	GCDFP-15
3.	52	.19	.957	GCDFP-15
4.	56	<.01	.993	CEA
5.	58	.07	.995	GCDFP-15
	89	.20	.956	CEA
6.	63	<.01	.987	GCDFP-15
7.	52	<.01	.989	GCDFP-15
	84	<.01	.965	CEA
8.	78	.30	.891	CEA
9.	79	<.01	.999	CEA
10.	69	.10	.988	GCDFP-15
	85	.014	.999	CEA
11.	124	.015	.981	GCDFP-15
12.	141	<.01	.987	GCDFP-15
13.	157	.25	.931	GCDFP-15
14.	174	.04	.956	CEA
	199	<.01	.993	GCDFP-15
15.	213	<.01	.987	CEA
16.	247	.011	.985	CEA

Of importance is the number of doublings in tumor marker level which occurred prior to clinical detection of metastasis. Listed in Tables 5 and 6, respectively, are the GCDFP-15 and CEA plasma levels which were attained by the time of clinical detection of metastasis. The number of doublings above the baseline abnormal marker value (GCDFP-15 >150 ng/ml and CEA >10 ng/ml) is tabulated in the second column of each table. For GCDFP-15 the maximum number of doublings observed was 5.53 and for CEA, 5.7. This number of doublings represents approximately a 50-fold increase in carcinoma volume during the disease-free interval if a 1:1 relationship between the circulating tumor marker level and carcinoma burden is assumed. Careful tumor-burden measurements of observable lesions vs. tumor marker levels are needed to validate this assumption.

Utilization of Plasma Markers for Monitoring Therapy in Metastatic Breast Carcinoma

Over the past four years 259 patients with metastatic breast carcinoma have been treated for their disease in the Breast

Table 5. GCDFP-15 Plasma Levels Attained by the Time of Clinical Detection of Metastasis

GCDFP-15 Level at Detection of Metastasis (ng/ml)	Calculated Number of Doublings >150 ng/ml	Observed* Log-Phase Doubling Time in Days	
6950	5.53	52	P < .01
6500	5.44	63	P < .01
1430	3.25	69	P .01
738	2.30		
711	2.24	58	P .07
673	2.17		
480	1.68	49	P .27
335	1.16	199	P < .01
330	1.14	141	P < .01
210	0.49	52	P .19
195	0.38		
178	0.25	124	P .015
177	0.25	157	P .25

*Includes GCDFP-15 levels below 150 ng/ml in calculation.

Table 6. CEA Plasma Levels Attained by the
Time of Clinical Detection of Metastasis

CEA Level at Detection of Metastasis (ng/ml)	Calculated Number of Doublings >10 ng/ml	Observed* Log-Phase Doubling Time in Days	
520	5.70	79	P <.01
52	2.38	85	P .014
52	2.38		
45	2.17	174	P .04
39	1.96	42	P .16
38	1.93	78	P .30
30	1.58	56	P <.01
29	1.54	84	P <.01
27	1.43	89	P .20
15	0.58		
14	0.49		
12	0.26	213	P <.01
12	0.26		
10	0.0	247	P .011

Oncology Clinic at Duke University Medical Center and have had serial CEA and GCDFP-15 plasma level determinations performed as part of the assessment of disease status. Slightly more than 4000 plasma samples have been analyzed. The longest duration of serial plasma marker level monitoring in a patient has been four years. The 259 patients are stratified in Table 7 relative to the predominant site of metastasis and the number of patients who have developed elevated plasma levels of GCDFP-15 only, CEA only, or both markers. Overall, 63% of the 259 patients have developed an elevated plasma marker level. The percentage of patients with elevated plasma marker levels was higher when osseous (71%) or viseral (64%) metastases were predominant, compared to soft tissue (36%) metastases. Of the 162 patients who developed elevated plasma marker levels, 82 (51%) had both markers elevated, while 49 (31%) had only CEA elevated and 31 (19%) had only GCDFP-15 elevated.

As metastatic breast carcinoma progresses, an increasing percentage of patients develop elevated plasma marker values.

Table 7. Metastatic Breast Carcinoma Patients

Predominant Location of Metastases	Number of Patients	GCDFP-15 >150 ng/ml Only	CEA >10 ng/ml Only	Both Markers Elevated	Total Markers Elevated
Soft tissue	47	5 (11%)	6 (13%)	6 (13%)	17 (36%)
Osseous	131	15 (11%)	20 (15%)	58 (44%)	93 (71%)
Visceral	81	11 (14%)	23 (28%)	18 (22%)	52 (64%)
Totals	259	31 (12%)	49 (19%)	82 (32%)	162 (63%)

In the group of 259 patients treated for metastatic disease, serial plasma marker levels were measured to within three months of death in 139 patients (Table 8). In this group 71% had developed elevated plasma levels of CEA and/or GCDFP-15. In contrast, of the 78 patients alive and currently being treated at Duke Medical Center, 47% had developed elevated plasma markers.

Also evident with progression of metastases is an increasing percentage of patients developing an elevation of both CEA and GCDFP-15. In Table 1 where metastatic disease was initially diagnosed, only 4 (17%) of the 23 patients with elevated markers had both markers elevated. In contrast, of the 139 patients followed to within three months of death (Table 8), 56 (56%) of the 99 with elevated plasma markers had both markers elevated.

The range of elevation in plasma marker level is an index of the degree of production of the plasma marker and also of the potential sensitivity of the marker to monitor metastatic disease

Table 8. Metastatic Breast Carcinoma Patients

Patient Category	Number of Patients	GCDFP-15 >150 ng/ml Only	CEA >10 ng/ml Only	Both Markers Elevated	Total Markers Elevated
Died	139	18 (13%)	25 (18%)	56 (40%)	99 (71%)
Alive	78	11 (14%)	13 (17%)	13 (17%)	34 (47%)
Lost to F/U*	42	2 (5%)	11 (26%)	13 (31%)	26 (62%)
Totals	259	31 (12%)	49 (19%)	82 (32%)	162 (63%)

*Lost to F/U = Patient no longer followed in the Breast Oncology Clinic at Duke Medical Center.

status. One hundred thirteen (44%) of the 259 patients with metastatic breast carcinoma (Fig. 3) had GCDFP-15 plasma levels above 150 ng/ml (range 150 ng/ml to 74,000 ng/ml), with 49 (19%) patients having values above 1000 ng/ml and 11 (4.2%) patients having values above 10,000 ng/ml. All patients with GCDFP-15 plasma values above 10,000 ng/ml had either osseous or visceral metastases predominant, as did 47 of the 49 patients above 1000 ng/ml. The highest observed GCDFP-15 value of 74,000 ng/ml represented approximately nine doublings in marker level above 150 ng/ml. This number of doublings correlates well with the range of up to ten doublings of breast carcinoma metastases expected between the time of clinical detection of metastases and death.

One hundred thirty-one (51%) of the 259 patients with metastatic breast carcinoma (Fig. 4) had CEA plasma levels above 10 ng/ml (range 10 ng/ml to 7000 ng/ml), with 43 (17%) patients above 100 ng/ml and 8 (3%) patients above 1000 ng/ml. All patients above 1000 ng/ml had either osseous or visceral metastases predominant, as did 41 of the 43 patients above 100 ng/ml. The highest observed CEA value of 7000 ng/ml represented approximately 9.5 doublings in marker level above 10 ng/ml. As with GCDFP-15, this number of CEA doublings encompasses the expected growth range of breast carcinoma metastases from the time of first clinical detection until death. Implied from the spectrum of CEA and GCDFP-15 plasma levels observed in metastatic breast carcinoma is that the higher plasma marker levels probably represent a combination of a larger tumor burden and an increased marker signal per cell (increased quantity of marker released per cell, or increased percentage of the total malignant cell population producing the marker).

Of the 259 patients with metastatic breast carcinoma, 100 had elevated plasma marker levels at the initiation of 151 treatments with five major forms of therapy utilized in the Breast Oncology Clinic at Duke Medical Center (Table 9). The patients are stratified relative to the number treated with each form of therapy, the direction of change in plasma marker level after initiation of therapy, and the duration of therapy.

The duration of therapy was chosen for evaluation rather than clinical response since therapy duration is an objective

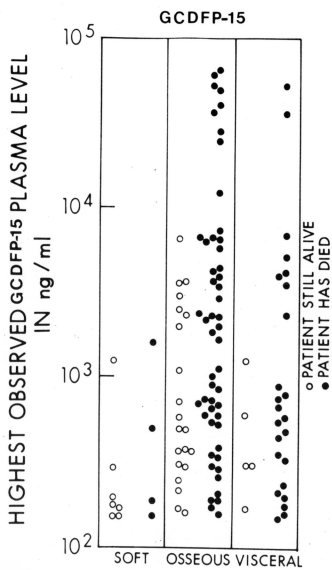

FIG. 3. Plot of the highest observed GCDFP-15 plasma level in ng/ml vs. the predominant location of breast carcinoma metastases. Eighty of the patients had died from metastatic disease and 33 were still alive at the time of analysis.

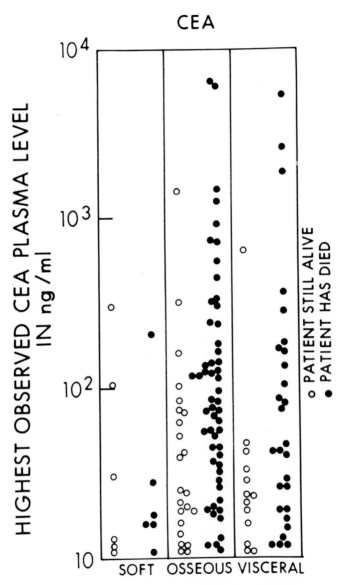

FIG. 4. Plot of the highest observed CEA plasma level in ng/ml vs. the predominant location of breast carcinoma metastases. Eighty-nine of the patients had died from metastatic disease and 42 were still alive at the time of analysis.

Table 9. Plasma Marker Profile Alterations Which Occurred with
151 Treatments Given for Metastatic Breast Carcinoma

Type of Therapy	No. of Patients	Direction Marker Change	Duration of Therapy		
			<3 Mo.	3-6 Mo.	>6 Mo.
Estrogen	27	Increase	4	1	0
		Stable	3	1	1
		Decrease	4	2	11
Tamoxifen	38	Increase	12	5	0
		Stable	5	6	3
		Decrease	0	4	3
Amino- glutethimide	24	Increase	4	3	1
		Stable	5	1	3
		Decrease	2	2	3
Cytoxan, 5-fluorouracil, methotrexate	26	Increase	1	1	1
		Stable	8	3	4
		Decrease	0	2	6
Adriamycin	36	Increase	2	1	2
		Stable	5	7	3
		Decrease	0	6	10
Totals	151	Increase	23	11	4
		Stable	26	18	14
		Decrease	6	16	33

measurement, whereas clinical response is to some degree subjective and has variability as to the criteria of assessment between physicians. The goal of therapy in metastatic breast carcinoma is palliation of disease symptoms. In this regard duration of a specific form of therapy is very important if the therapy is being effective for palliation.

An increasing plasma marker profile with initiation of therapy occurred in 38 patients. Only 4 (11%) of the 38 patients remained on therapy for over six months and 23 (61%) had therapy discontinued within three months. In contrast, of the 55 patients whose plasma marker levels decreased with initiation of therapy, only 6 (11%) were discontinued from therapy within three months and 33 (60%) remained on therapy for over six months.

Within the five categories of therapy evaluated, 26 (42%) of the 62 patients treated with chemotherapy were maintained on therapy for over six months. Sixteen (62%) of the 26 patients had an initial decrease in plasma marker levels, while 7 (27%) had stable levels and 3 (12%) had increasing levels.

Of the 27 patients given estrogen therapy, 12 (44%) were maintained on therapy for over six months, and 11 (92%) of the 12 had an initial decrease in plasma marker level while 1 (8%) remained stable. Of the 38 patients treated with tamoxifen, 6 (16%) were maintained on therapy for over six months, with 3 of the 6 having an initial decrease in plasma marker level and 3 remaining stable.

Of the 24 patients treated with aminoglutethimide (1000 mg daily with 10 mg hydrocortisone four times a day), 7 (29%) were maintained on therapy for over six months. Three of these 7 patients had initial decreases in plasma marker levels, while 3 remained stable and 1 elevated.

The time interval to a 50% decrease in plasma marker level was analyzed for each of the five treatment groups (Fig. 5). Hormonal therapy induced a more rapid 50% decrease in plasma marker level (average for estrogen and tamoxifen therapy — 24 days) than did chemotherapy (average 65 days). No patient initially given chemotherapy had a 50% decrease in marker level during the first three weeks. In contrast, for estrogen and tamoxifen therapy, half of the 50% decreases in plasma marker levels had occurred by three weeks and 100% had occurred by eight weeks.

The difference in the time frame to a 50% decrease in plasma marker level with initiation of hormonal vs. chemical therapy is of interest relative to the mechanism of action of the various drugs on cancer cells, as well as being important clinically with regard to the time frame necessary for assessment of response to therapy utilizing plasma markers.

Effective hormonal therapy for metastatic breast carcinoma with estrogen or tamoxifen appears to cause the inhibition in synthesis of CEA and GCDFP-15 quickly, and the plasma levels of these two proteins decrease, in general, ahead of overt clinical signs of response to therapy. In contrast, chemical therapy with either adriamycin or Cytoxan, 5-fluorouracil and methotrexate appears to require several cycles of therapy before decreasing plasma levels of CEA and GCDFP-15 occur, and the time frame of clinical assessment of response to therapy usually coincides with the marker level alterations.

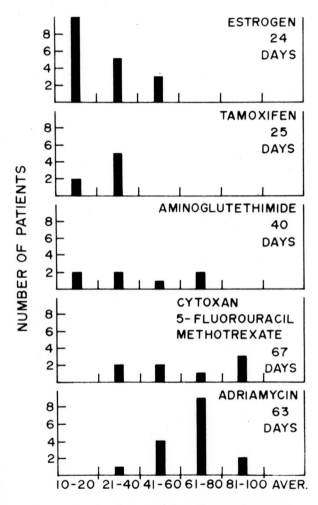

HISTOGRAM OF TIME INTERVAL
UNTIL A 50% DECREASE IN
PLASMA MARKER LEVEL

DAYS TO 50% DECREASE IN MARKER LEVEL

FIG. 5. Histogram of time interval until a 50% decrease in plasma marker level occurred after initiation of therapy.

One explanation for the differences observed in the time frame of plasma marker response to chemical vs. hormonal therapy is that hormonal therapy directly poisons the protein synthetic apparatus of the breast carcinoma cell (probably by direct inhibition of the M-RNA synthesis signal), whereas chemical therapy is mainly directed at DNA synthesis and inhibits protein synthesis only secondarily.

Another question concerning tumor markers is whether their production rate or release from carcinoma cells can be enhanced with a specific stimulus. An example of a specific stimulus for a tumor marker is the induced release of calcitonin from medullary carcinoma of the thyroid by injection of calcium and pentagrastrin into the systemic circulation [30]. Carcinoma cell CEA production has not been demonstrated to be enhanced by any specific stimulus. In medullary carcinoma of the thyroid the stimulus which releases calcitonin has no effect on circulating CEA level [31].

Human breast gross cystic disease is a premenopausal disease in women and it is probably induced by either an imbalance in hormonal stimulus to the breast or response by breast cells to hormones. In this regard the constituent proteins produced in gross cystic disease fluid can be considered to be hormonally induced. The potential thus exists for the GCDFP-15 protein produced by breast carcinoma cells to be hormonally modulated. Our clinical observations on treatment of metastatic breast carcinoma patients with Halotestin have indicated that the GCDFP-15 plasma levels rapidly elevate two- to three-fold on initiation of this therapy in approximately one third of the treated patients (Fig. 6). This change in GCDFP-15 plasma level did not correlate with an objective change in disease status and the rate of increase was too rapid to reflect tumor doubling. Our hypothesis is that Halotestin therapy increases the production of GCDFP-15 in the carcinoma cells. The CEA plasma levels in the same patient did not demonstrate any significant change within the same four-week time frame (Fig. 7). Since only a proportion of the patients given Halotestin had GCDFP-15 plasma levels increase greater than 100% in four weeks, this indicates variation in the induction effect. The opposite effect of a drop in GCDFP-15 plasma level with discontinuation of Halotestin therapy has also been observed.

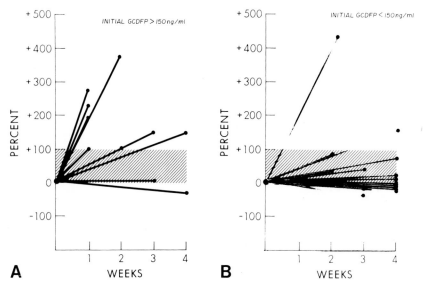

FIG. 6. Percentage of change in GCDFP-15 plasma level with initiation of Halotestin therapy. (A) Patients with initial GCDFP-15 >150 ng/ml. (B) Patients with initial GCDFP-15 <150 ng/ml.

Further observations are required to more precisely define the effect of Halotestin and related steroids on GCDFP-15 production in breast carcinoma cells. It will also be important to correlate this GCDFP-15 modulation with other parameters of hormonal sensitivity of breast carcinoma cells. With regard to clinical treatment, when Halotestin is added to other forms of therapy for breast carcinoma, a time frame of two to four weeks is required to define the "stimulated" baseline level of GCDFP-15; also, when Halotestin is discontinued, the non-stimulated GCDFP-15 baseline will require a two- to four-week interval to become established.

Conclusion

Biological markers of breast carcinoma are important substances which can aid in our understanding of the pathophysiology of this disease, serve as monitors of disease status and potentially be utilized as a point of attack for therapy. A summary of our findings on utilization of plasma markers to

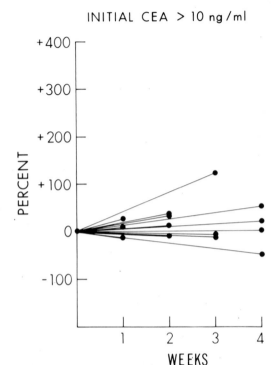

FIG. 7. Percentage of change in CEA level with initiation of Halotestin therapy.

detect and monitor therapy for metastatic breast carcinoma is presented below:

1. Approximately 25% of the postmastectomy patients who developed recurrence of breast carcinoma had elevated plasma levels of GCDFP-15 and/or CEA for 21 to 693 days (average 210 days) prior to any other objective signs of recurrence.

2. Logarithmically increasing plasma marker profiles were observed in most cases once the plasma marker level became distinctly abnormal (CEA >10 ng/ml and GCDFP-15 >150 ng/ml). The doubling time of the logarithmically increasing marker profiles was from 42 to 247 days, with a mean time of 106 days. All marker profiles with logarithmically increasing values continued

to elevate until clinical detection of metastasis and institution of therapy.

3. Approximately 70% of patients with metastatic breast carcinoma developed elevated plasma levels of CEA and/or GCDFP-15 by the time of death. Half of the patients with elevated marker levels had both CEA and GCDFP-15 elevated, while 30% had only CEA and 20% had only GCDFP-15 elevated.

4. The direction of change in the plasma marker level correlated with the duration of therapy. Decreasing levels were associated with therapy duration for more than six months in >60% of treated patients. In contrast, increasing values were associated with discontinuation of therapy in less than three months in >60% of treated patients.

5. The time frame for a greater than 50% reduction in plasma marker level after initiation of therapy was dependent upon the type of therapy given. For estrogen or tamoxifen therapy the CEA and GCDFP-15 plasma level decreases of greater than 50% all occurred within eight weeks, and over half of the decreases occurred within three weeks. In contrast, the greater than 50% decreases of plasma markers with effective chemotherapy were slower to occur and only approximately half had occurred by eight weeks.

6. The GCDFP-15 molecule appeared to be hormonally modulated to some degree by Halotestin, and initiation of this therapy induced increased plasma levels of GCDFP-15 without an alteration in disease status. The time frame of observed increased plasma levels was two to four weeks. Thus, whenever Halotestin or other androgens are given, a two- to four-week period is necessary to establish a new "stimulated" GCDFP-15 baseline before determining direction of marker change. The same time frame is necessary for establishing the nonstimulated GCDFP-15 baseline when Halotestin is discontinued.

7. A conservative set of criteria for determining response to therapy with alteration in plasma marker profiles would be the following:

(a) Plasma marker levels need to be definitively abnormal at start of therapy (CEA >10 ng/ml and GCDFP-15 >150 ng/ml).
(b) The serial trend in the plasma marker level is critical to proper assessment.
(c) Serial values should be obtained at monthly intervals.
(d) Increasing values >100% are indicative of progression.
(e) Decreasing values greater than 50% are indicative of regression.

References

1. Ip, C. and Dao, T.: Alteration in serum glycosyltransferases and 5'-nucleotidases in breast cancer patients. Cancer Res. 38:723-728, 1978.
2. Ehrmeyer, S.L., Joiner, B.L., Kahan, L. et al: A cancer associated fast homoarginine-sensitive electrophoretic form of serum alkaline phosphatase. Cancer Res. 38:599-601, 1978.
3. Marcus, D.M. and Zinberg, N.: Measurement of serum ferritin by radioimmunoassay: Results in normal individuals and patients with breast cancer. JNCI 55:791-795, 1975.
4. Springer, G.F., Desai, P.R. and Banatwala, I.: Blood group MN antigens and precursors in normal and malignant human breast glandular tissue. JNCI 34:335-339, 1975.
5. Grosser, N. and Thomson, D.M.P.: Cell-mediated antitumor immunity in breast cancer patients evaluated by antigen-induced leukocyte adherence inhibition in test tubes. Cancer Res. 35:2571-2579, 1975.
6. LoGerfo, P., Krupey, J. and Hansen, H.J.: Demonstration of an antigen common to several varieties of neoplasia. Assay using zirconyl phosphate gel. N. Engl. J. Med. 285:138-141, 1971.
7. Chu, T.M. and Nemoto, T.: Evaluation of carcinoembryonic antigen in human mammary carcinoma. JNCI 51:1119-1122, 1973.
8. Laurence, D.J.R., Stevens, U., Bettelheim, R. et al: Role of plasma carcinoembryonic antigen in diagnosis of gastrointestinal, mammary, and bronchial carcinoma. Br. Med. J. 3:605-609, 1972.
9. Steward, A.M., Nixon, D., Zamcheck, N. and Aisenberg, A.: Carcinoembryonic antigen in breast cancer patients. Serum levels and disease progress. Cancer 33:1246-1252, 1974.
10. Tormey, D.C., Waalkes, T.P. and Simon, R.M.: Biological markers in breast carcinoma. II. Clinical correlations with human chorionic gonadotrophin. Cancer 39:2391-2396, 1977.
11. Sheth, N.A., Suraiya, J.N., Sheth, A.R. et al: Ectopic production of human placental lactogen by human breast tumors. Cancer 39:1693-1699, 1977.

12. Franchimont, P., Zangerle, P.F., Hendrick, J.C. et al: Simultaneous assays of cancer associated antigens in benign and malignant breast diseases (CEA, alpha fetal protein, HCG, K-casein). Cancer 39:2806-2812, 1977.
13. Hendrick, J.C. and Franchimont, P.: Radioimmunoassay of casein in the serum of normal subjects and patients with various malignancies. Eur. J. Cancer 10:725-730, 1974.
14. Kleinberg, D.L.: Human α-lactalbumin. Measurement in serum and in breast cancer organ cultures by radioimmunoassay. Science 190:276-278, 1975.
15. Haagensen, D.E., Jr., Mazoujian, G., Holder, W.D. et al: Evaluation of a breast cyst fluid protein detectable in the plasma of breast carcinoma patients. Ann. Surg. 187:277-285, 1977.
16. Gold, P. and Freedman, S.O.: Demonstration of tumor-specific antigens in human colonic carcinomata by immunological tolerance and absorption techniques. J. Exp. Med. 121:439-462, 1965.
17. Gold, P. and Freedman, S.O.: Specific carcinoembryonic antigens of the human digestive system. J. Exp. Med. 122:467-481, 1965.
18. Hansen, H.J., Lance, K.P. and Krupey, J.: Demonstration of an ion-sensitive antigenic site on carcinoembryonic antigen using zirconyl phosphate gel. Clin. Res. 19:143, 1971.
19. Hansen, H.J., Hager, H.J., Cohen, H. et al: Induction of an antisera monospecific for carcinoembryonic antigen. Clin. Res. 19:53, 1971.
20. Haagensen, D.E., Jr., Kister, S.J., Vandevoorde, J.P. et al: Evaluation of carcinoembryonic antigen as a plasma monitor for human breast carcinoma. Cancer 42:1512-1519, 1978.
21. Thomson, D.M.P., Krupey, J., Freedman, S.O. and Gold, P.: The radioimmunoassay of circulating carcinoembryonic antigen of the human digestive system. Proc. Natl. Acad. Sci. U.S.A. 64:161-167, 1969.
22. Hansen, H.J., Snyder, J.J., Miller, E. et al: Carcinoembryonic antigen (CEA) assay, a laboratory adjunct in the diagnosis and management of cancer. Hum. Pathol. 5:139-147, 1974.
23. Kupchik, H.Z., Loewenstein, M.S., Feil, M. et al: The disparity of indirect and direct zirconyl-gel analysis for carcinoembryonic antigen. Cancer 42:1589-1594, 1978.
24. Haagensen, D.E., Jr., Easterday, R.L., Stolle, C.A. and Wells, S.A., Jr.: Buffer-exchange column for rapid separating of carcinoembryonic antigen from perchloric acid. Clin. Chem. 24:135-137, 1978.
25. Haagensen, D.E., Jr., Mazoujian, G., Dilley, W.G. et al: Breast gross cystic disease fluid analysis. I. Isolation and radioimmunoassay for a major component protein. JNCI 62:239-247, 1979.
26. Haagensen, D.E., Jr., Kister, S.J., Panick, J. et al: Comparative evaluation of carcinoembryonic antigen and gross cystic disease fluid protein as plasma markers for human breast carcinoma. Cancer 42:1646-1652, 1978.
27. Haagensen, D.E., Jr. and Wells, S.A., Jr.: Plasma human breast gross cystic disease fluid assay. In Herberman, R.B. (ed.): Compendium of

Assays for Immunodiagnosis of Human Cancer. New York:Elsevier-North Holland Publishing Co., 1979, pp. 397-405.

28. Philippe, F. and Le Gal, Y.: Growth of seventy-eight recurrent mammary cancers. Cancer 21:461-467, 1968.

29. Collins, V.P., Loeffler, R.K. and Tivey, H.: Observations on growth rates of human tumors. Am. J. Roentgenol. Rad. Ther. Nucl. Med. 76:988-1000, 1956.

30. Wells, S.A., Jr., Baylin, S.B., Linehan, W.M. et al: Provocative agents and the diagnosis of medullary carcinoma of the thyroid gland. Ann. Surg. 188:139-141, 1978.

31. Wells, S.A., Jr., Haagensen, D.E., Jr., Linehan, W.M. et al: The detection of elevated plasma levels of carcinoembryonic antigen in patients with suspected or established medullary thyroid carcinoma. Cancer 42:1498-1503, 1978.

Self-Evaluation Quiz

1. In any assay the higher the abnormal level is set, the greater the specificity and the poorer the sensitivity.
   a) True
   b) False

2. Abnormal CEA levels have been defined as >2.5 ng/ml to >10.0 ng/ml.
   a) True
   b) False

3. All changes in CEA levels in serial measurements correlate closely with changes in disease status.
   a) True
   b) False

4. A normal plasma range of GCDFP-15 has been established at:
   a) 9 to 30 ng/ml
   b) 30 to 80 ng/ml
   c) 0 to 50 ng/ml
   d) 0 to 80 ng/ml

5. All major forms of malignancy in women demonstrate plasma elevations of GCDFP-15 above 150 ng/ml.
   a) True
   b) False

6. With progression of metastases there is an increasing percentage of patients with an elevation of both CEA and GCDFP-15.

a) True
b) False
7. Effective chemotherapy for metastatic breast carcinoma inhibits synthesis of both markers, and plasma levels decrease before overt clinical signs of response to therapy.
a) True
b) False
8. Chemical therapy is directed mainly at:
a) Protein synthesis
b) M-RNA synthesis
c) DNA synthesis

Answers on page 335.

Phantom Breast Sensation Following Mastectomy for Malignant Breast Disease

Gordon F. Schwartz, M.D. and Harry M. Rosenblum, M.D.

Objectives

The occurrence of phantom breast sensation following mastectomy for cancer has been described infrequently in the medical literature. The purpose of this paper is to present an analysis of detailed questionnaires received from 79 of 155 queried patients who had undergone mastectomy — in order to ascertain the incidence of these phantom breast sensations and to identify the clinical situations in which this phenomenon might be expected.

Phantom pain and similar sensations are well-known sequelae of extremity amputations; less well known are similar phenomena following mastectomy. Nevertheless, phantom breast sensation may be considered a distinct clinical entity, and has been reported in as many as 64% of women undergoing mastectomy. A definition of phantom breast sensation is difficult, but it is best described as a feeling which seems to emanate from the area of the resected breast, as though it were still present. The sensation may be one that itches, burns, tingles, twists, pulls or feels like "pins and needles." No etiology has been elucidated. Reported variables which have been alleged to correlate with the presence of phantom breast sensations include its prevalence among younger patients, premenopausal patients, those who experience postoperative edema of the arm

Gordon F. Schwartz, M.D., F.A.C.S., Professor of Surgery, Jefferson Medical College; Director of Clinical Services, Breast Diagnostic Center; and Harry M. Rosenblum, M.D., Resident Surgeon, Thomas Jefferson University Hospital, Philadelphia, Pa.

and patients who suffer a significant degree of postmastectomy depression [1]. More recently, it has been stated that women who experience phantom pain also are more critical of the emotional support received from their surgeons before, during and after the operative procedure [2]. This present study was undertaken to ascertain the incidence of postmastectomy phantom breast sensations and to attempt to identify those clinical situations in which this phenomenon might be expected.

Methods

Detailed questionnaires were sent to 155 patients who had undergone either radical, modified radical or total mastectomy for the treatment of carcinoma of the breast. All of the patients came from a single surgical practice, and 98% of the patients had been operated on by the same surgeon (G.F.S.). Length of time between mastectomy and this query ranged from two months to 15 years. The questionnaire contained 51 items, including type of mastectomy, occurrence of postoperative complications, evaluation of physician support, evaluation of support given by spouse or lover, presence of perioperative depression, body image and an extensive section questioning the occurrence of phantom sensations. This latter section included questions asking specifically for different types of sensations which might be encountered, their frequency, location, length of duration, initiating factors and the extent of the interference of these symptoms with daily activities. Wording for each item required only that the patient check the appropriate response, but space was also provided for written comments. Signatures were optional. No specific psychological testing was performed.

Results

Seventy-nine complete responses had been received as of August 1, 1979, and constitute the data upon which this report is based. The age of the patients at the time of mastectomy ranged from 34 to 71 years, the mean being 54. The 79 responses were divided into two groups: group A, those who described any phantom sensations, and group B, those patients denying the presence of any such sensations (Table 1). Group A comprised 48 of the 79 patients, or 60.8%; group B, 31 patients

Table 1. Analysis of Responses from 79 Mastectomy Patients

	Group A (Symptoms)	Group B (No Symptoms)
Number of Patients	48 (60.8%)	31 (39.2%)
Mean Age	55.7	52.3
Married	32 (66.6%)	23 (74.2%)
Premenopausal	10 (20.8%)	7 (22.6%)
Emotional Adjustment Good to excellent	40 (83.3%)	26 (83.9%)
Surgeon Support Good to excellent	46 (95.8%)	31 (100%)
Husband Support Good to excellent	30 (62.5%)	25 (80.6%)
Poor	9 (18.8%)	1 (3.2%)

or 39.2%. Of those patients in group A, all of whom described phantom sensations, 24 (50%) considered these sensations "uncomfortable" at some time. The mean ages of the patients in both groups were similar, 56 years for patients with symptoms and 52 years for patients without. Most patients in both groups were married, and approximately the same number in each group were premenopausal. Ninety-six percent of the patients who experienced any phantom sensations felt their surgeon's support was good to excellent; all of the patients in the group without symptoms said the same. Support from spouse or lover was considered poor in 18.8% of those patients with phantom sensations but in only 3.2% of those patients without. Other factors which pertain to personal emotional adjustments, such as body image, were about equal in both groups; 85.3% in the affected group and 83.9% in the unaffected group considered their own adjustment as "satisfactory" or better.

Words used by the patients to describe the sensations experienced included terms such as itching, burning, tingling, twisting, pulling, sticking and a "pins and needles" feeling. Two patients described their sensations as pleasant, even erotic ones. There was no consistency in the duration of the sensations, which ranged from seconds only to a continual presence of the sensation. There was no specific precipitating factor noted.

Sometimes the sensation was initiated by physical activity or changes in weather. A majority of the patients felt that their phantom sensation arose spontaneously. The area of the absent breast from which the sensations seemed to emanate was the entire breast in 45.8% of the patients. Nipple and/or areola seemed to be present and symptomatic in 18.8% of the patients. The only quadrant of the breast mentioned significantly was that of the upper outer quadrant in 14.6% of the patients. The other three quadrants of the breast sere described much less frequently, but the descriptions of the origin of the sensation correlated well with the location of the primary tumor.

Of the entire group of 79 patients responding to the questionnaire, 21 (26.6%) experienced what was not considered to be phantom sensation but, rather, an uncomfortable or annoying feeling in the wound when they drank hot or cold liquids. This hot or cold feeling seemed to radiate from the posterior pharynx down across the chest and into the operative site. This particular sensation lasted only seconds and only occurred when the patients drank very warm or very cold liquids.

The following items about which specific questions were asked did not seem to correlate with the phantom sensations: type of mastectomy, i.e. radical, modified radical, etc.; presence or absence of skin graft; race; religion; postoperative chemotherapy or radiation therapy; postoperative wound infection; postoperative wound drainage (seroma); arm swelling; menstrual history or menopausal symptoms; age; previous or present feeling of depression; personal concept of body image.

Discussion

Phantom limb pain subsequent to amputation of an extremity was noted in the 16th century by Ambroise Paré [3], but the classical description of phantom sensation was made in the 19th century by S. Weir Mitchell [4], who recorded the existence of phantom breast sensation as well. Crone-Muzerbrock [5] reported a clinical study of phantom breast sensation in 1950, observing these symptoms in 53% of 49 patients who had undergone mastectomy. Ackerley et al [6] noted an incidence of 22% of phantom breast sensations and remarked that patients with these sensations tended to be younger than those who did not experience them. This finding relating age to phantom breast sensations was confirmed by Jarvis [1] in a study of 104 patients with a 23% incidence of phantom breast. Jarvis also noted that premenopausal mastectomy was more likely to be associated with phantom breast.

The descriptions of the sensations felt by patients experiencing phantom breast are similar to those known to occur in limb amputees [7]. Most commonly, there is only an awareness of the entire breast being present or a mild tingling feeling at that site. Many other sensations have also been described, but actual pain or discomfort is the most annoying of the symptoms, reported in between 18% and 80% of mastectomy patients [1, 2, 5, 6, 8, 9].

This present report documents a high incidence of phantom breast sensation, an overall incidence of 60.8% of the patients returning the questionnaire. Fifty percent of the patients reported that their symptoms were at some time uncomfortable, but no patients described a significant degree of discomfort and no patient's daily activities were affected by the sensations. As previously noted, two patients described the sensations as pleasant, even mildly erotic. An unusual sensation which has not been reported previously was noted by 21 of the patients in this study. This feeling was a sensation of heat or cold radiating into the operative site on the chest wall at the time of swallowing a hot or cold drink, respectively. This sensation was fleeting and never lasted more than a few seconds.

This study did not demonstrate any significant correlation between postmastectomy depression and the occurrence of phantom breast sensations. More than 80% of the patients who had phantom breast sensations reported that their adjustment to life after their mastectomy was good to excellent, and they were able to resume most or all of the activities that they performed prior to mastectomy.

Unlike previous reports [1, 2, 6], this study did not demonstrate a significant age difference between those patients with and without phantom breast sensations. Similarly, menopausal status did not correlate with the occurrence of phantom breast. These findings contrast with prior reports [1, 2, 6] which suggested that the younger premenopausal patient is at higher risk for this phenomenon. Other variables not demon-

strated to be of significance were postoperative wound complications, arm edema, adjuvant chemotherapy or radiation
therapy, type of mastectomy and personal feelings of body
image.

In a recent study by Jamison et al [2], women experiencing
phantom breast sensations seemed to be more critical of their
relationship with their lover or spouse, of the emotional support
received from their surgeon and of their overall emotional
adjustments after mastectomy. A relationship between the last
two variables and phantom breast sensations was not supported
by this study. Of the 48 patients who reported phantom breast
symptoms, 96% noted that the surgical support received pre-
and post-operatively was good to excellent, and 83.3% of these
patients felt themselves to be well adjusted emotionally. This
seems to indicate that the surgeon's support, although obviously
of prime importance, has no direct bearing on the development
of phantom breast sensations. Also, these symptoms seemed to
occur just as frequently in the well-adjusted patients as in the
depressed or emotionally upset individuals.

The only significant variable noted in this study which
correlated with phantom breast sensation is that of spouse or
lover support. This finding is consistent with the report by
Jamison et al [2]. Of those women who described any phantom
breast sensations, 18.8% thought the support provided by their
spouse or lover before, during or after the mastectomy was
poor; of the women who did not experience this phenomenon,
only 3.2% had the same feelings of abandonment. This supports
the suggestion that it is the patient's relationship to her spouse
or lover which is a more important factor than the surgeon's
emotional support in the period surrounding mastectomy.

This documentation that some phantom breast sensations
occur in a majority of patients who have undergone mastectomy for malignant disease implies that this should be an item
of discussion with a patient facing the prospect of mastectomy.
Although the phantom breast syndrome, when it does occur, is
not particularly uncomfortable, its very presence may be
discomforting to the patient and a cause for alarm. Discussing
the possibility of this symptom complex occurring makes it
much less likely to be of consequence.

The apparent correlation between lack of emotional support
by husband or lover and the occurrence of postmastectomy

phantom breast sensation is also noteworthy. Obviously, maximum emotional support should be offered by all of the patient's family, friends and physicians. The occurrence of phantom breast sensations is only one manifestation of a deficiency in this area.

Summary

More than 60% of 79 patients who had undergone some form of mastectomy as treatment for carcinoma of the breast experienced phantom breast sensations in the postoperative period. This high proportion of women who experienced this phenomenon is notable. The presence or absence of these symptoms did not seem to correlate with patient's age, race, religion, type of mastectomy performed, need for adjuvant chemotherapy or radiation therapy, presence of postoperative infection, seroma or the patient's perceptions of her own adjustment to her mastectomy. Almost all patients, even those who experienced this syndrome, described good to excellent rapport with the operating surgeon. The only variable which seemed to be of significance was the presence or absence of emotional support of husband or lover at the time of surgery or postmastectomy. Patients who described their support from husband or lover as poor were much more likely to experience these sensations than were women whose emotional support was described as good or excellent.

References

1. Jarvis, J.H.: Post-mastectomy breast phantoms. J. Nerv. Ment. Dis. 144:266-272, 1967.
2. Jamison, D., Wellisch, D.K., Katz, R.L. and Pasnau, R.O.: Phantom breast syndrome. Arch. Surg. 144:93-95, 1979.
3. Paré, A.: Oeuvres Completes, J. F. Malgaigne, ed. Paris: 1840, vol. 2, pp. 221-231.
4. Mitchell, S.W.: Phantom limbs. Mag. Popular Lit. Sci. Educ. 8:563, Dec. 1871.
5. Crone-Muzerbrock, A.: Phantomjefuhle und Phantomschmerz vach Mammamputation. Langenbecks Arch. Clin. Chir. 266:569-575, 1950.
6. Ackerley, W., Lhamon, W. and Fitto, W.T.: Phantom breast. J. Nerv. Ment. Dis. 121:143-151, 1955.
7. Hoffman, J.: Phantom ·limb syndrome. J. Nerv. Ment. Dis. 122:143-151, 1955.
8. Simmel, M.L.: A study of phantoms after amputation of the breast. Neuropsychologia 4:331-350, 1966.

9. Weinstein, S., Vetter, R.J. and Sersen, E.A.: Phantoms following breast amputation. Neuropsychologia 8:185-197, 1970.

Self-Evaluation Quiz

1. Phantom breast sensations are rare following mastectomy for cancer.
   a) True
   b) False
2. The patients most likely to experience these sensations after mastectomy include:
   a) Women whose support from husband is considered poor
   b) Women who have had radical mastectomy
   c) Women who have had a postoperative wound infection
   d) Women who are premenopausal
   e) All of the above
3. The proportion of women experiencing phantom breast sensations following mastectomy is:
   a) 10%
   b) 20%
   c) 40%
   d) 60%
   e) 80%
4. The patient's own perceptions of her body image are very important in determining whether she is likely to experience phantom breast sensations after mastectomy.
   a) True
   b) False
5. The phantom breast sensations described by patients are uniformly unpleasant and uncomfortable sensations.

   a) True
   b) False

Answers on page 335.

Answers to Self-Evaluation Quizzes

Page 18:   1(d); 2(e); 3(d); 4(d); 5(b); 6(e); 7(b); 8(a); 9(b); 10(c); 11(d); 12(a); 13(e); 14(c); 15(c).

Page 29:   1(b); 2(a); 3(e); 4(d); 5(b); 6(e); 7(c); 8(c).

Page 40:   1(b); 2(a); 3(a); 4(c); 5(d); 6(d); 7(c); 8(b); 9(d); 10(d).

Page 52:   1(b); 2(c); 3(b); 4(c); 5(a); 6(b); 7(d); 8(b); 9(a); 10(c); 11(c); 12(d); 13(a); 14(f); 15(b).

Page 65:   1(b); 2(a); 3(a); 4(b); 5(a); 6(c); 7(c); 8(c); 9(b); 10(d).

Page 70:   1(a); 2(c); 3(b); 4(a).

Page 84:   1(a); 2(a); 3(a); 4(a); 5(a); 6(a); 7(a); 8(a).

Page 96:   1(d,e); 2(c); 3(d); 4(a); 5(a); 6(a); 7(d); 8(a); 9(a); 10(a); 11(a); 12(a); 13(a).

Page 107:   1(b); 2(c); 3(a); 4(d); 5(b); 6(c).

Page 121:   1(a); 2(d); 3(b); 4(a); 5(a); 6(a); 7(a); 8(a); 9(a); 10(a).

Page 135:   1(b);   2(b);   3(a);   4(a);   5(b);   6(c);   7(a,b); 8(a,b,c,d,e); 9(a,c); 10(c,d).

Page 142:   1(b); 2(a); 3(a); 4(d); 5(b); 6(c); 7(a).

Page 148:   1(a); 2(a); 3(a); 4(a); 5(a); 6(a).

Page 172:   1(a); 2(a); 3(a); 4(b); 5(a); 6(a); 7(b,c,a).

Page 179:   1(a); 2(b); 3(a); 4(d); 5(b).

Page 202:   1(e); 2(d); 3(c); 4(a); 5(a); 6(c); 7(a); 8(c); 9(a); 10(a); 11(c); 12(a); 13(a); 14(d).

Page 213:   1(a); 2(b); 3(b); 4(a); 5(a); 6(a); 7(d); 8(b); 9(a); 10(a).

Page 236:   1(b); 2(b); 3(b); 4(b); 5(a).

Page 248:   1(b); 2(c); 3(b); 4(b); 5(d); 6(b); 7(b); 8(d); 9(b); 10(b).

Page 273:   1(d); 1(b); 3(b); 4(c); 5(a); 6(a); 7(c); 8(d); 9(c); 10(c).

Page 287:   1(d); 2(a); 3(c); 4(b); 5(e); 6(a).

Page 299:   1(b); 2(b); 3(b); 4(b); 5(b).

Page 324:   1(a); 2(a); 3(b); 4(d); 5(b); 6(a); 7(b); 8(c).

Page 334:   1(b); 2(a); 3(d); 4(b); 5(b).

Subject Index

WP 840 B74 1980
Breast diseas   nlm

3 0081 004 229 237